falls in older people

falls in older people

prevention and management

third edition

by

rein tideiksaar, Ph.D.

HEALTH PROFESSIONS PRESS

Baltimore • London • Winnipeg • Sydney

HEALTH PROFESSIONS PRESS

Health Professions Press, Inc.
Post Office Box 10624
Baltimore, MD 21285-0624
www.healthpropress.com

Typeset by Barton Matheson Willse & Worthington, Baltimore, Maryland.
Manufactured in the United States of America by Versa Press, Inc., East Peoria, Illinois.

Illustrations by Juanita Wassenaar-Beggs.

All of the case studies in this book are composites of the author's actual experiences. In all instances, names have been changed; in some instances, identifying details have been altered to protect confidentiality.

Library of Congress Cataloging-in-Publication Data

Tideiksaar, Rein.
    Falls in older persons : prevention and management / Tideiksaar.—3rd ed.
      p.   cm.
    Includes bibliographical references and index.
    ISBN 1-878812-85-8
    1. Falls (Accidents) in old age.   2. Falls (Accidents) in old age—Prevention. 3. Aged—Hospital Care.   4. Aged—Nursing home care.
I. Title.
RC952.5 .T53 2002
617.1'0084'6—dc21

                                      2002068638

British Library of Cataloguing in Publication data are available from the British Library.

contents

about the author

Rein Tideiksaar, Ph.D., is Senior Vice President of Fall Prevention Services, Strategies and Technologies, Eldercare Companies, Inc., in Philadelphia, Pennsylvania; and Chairman of the Science, Technology, and Resource Task Force of the National Alliance to Prevent Falls As We Age. From 1996 to 2000, Dr. Tideiksaar was the Director of Geriatric Educational and Clinical Programs, Southwest Medical Associates, Sierra Health Services, Inc., in Las Vegas, Nevada. Prior to 1996, he was Director of Falls and Immobility Programs, Henry L. Schwartz Department of Geriatrics, Mount Sinai Medical Center, in New York, New York.

Dr. Tideiksaar obtained a doctorate from Columbia Pacific University and a physician assistant certification from the State University of New York at Stony Brook. Dr. Tideiksaar completed his geriatric training at the Parker Jewish Geriatric Institute, New Hyde Park, New York.

In addition to two previous editions of this professional resource, Dr. Tideiksaar has written numerous articles and book chapters and the textbook, *Falling in Old Age, Second Edition* (Springer Publishing, 1997), on the topic of falls in older adults. He has conducted fall-related research and developed fall prevention programs in communities, acute care hospitals, and nursing facilities.

preface to
the third edition

While I was writing the third edition of *Falls in Older People*, several things became readily evident to me. First, although falls in acute care hospitals and nursing facilities continue to be a serious problem, interest in fall prevention has never been stronger. Acute care hospitals and nursing facilities are devoting a great deal of attention toward developing fall prevention programs. One reason for this is that most hospital and nursing-facility providers have been successful at eliminating restraints (a practice quite common until the 1990s). Although restraint reduction is certainly a more humane tendency in these care facilities, a by-product is, in many instances, an increase in falls.

Second, as I visit hospitals and nursing facilities it is apparent to me that busy clinicians require simple and straightforward approaches to managing the problem of falls. In an effort to help these organizations and clinicians, the aim of the third edition remains the same—to educate acute care hospital and nursing facility health professionals about falls. It is my firm belief that if organizations and professionals are knowledgeable about what causes falls and how to prevent them, then the risk of falling can be greatly minimized.

Third, I've begun to recognize the fact that for many health professionals, falling is a complex problem to solve. Previous editions, which were titled *Falls in Older Persons*, have been praised by several professional organizations and have received numerous awards. This kind of attention always makes an author feel good. But the most rewarding feedback I get comes from health professionals working in the field who have told me on numerous occasions how useful the book has been in their fall prevention activities and efforts. Therefore, at least to a certain extent, I believe that I've been successful in making the topic of falls easy to understand for many health professionals.

This third edition, now titled *Falls in Older People*, continues this easy-to-understand style of writing. In addition to updating the chapters, bibliography, and case study exercises, I've included new guidelines and forms for helping hospital and nursing facility professionals develop their fall prevention programs through best practices. Because fall risk assessments, restraints, bed safety, siderails and fall/restraint-use rate calculations are of topical interest, I've included guidelines on these issues. It is my hope that this book will be read from cover to cover until its pages are worn thin through repeated readings. That will mean that I've continued to be successful in making the problem of falls understandable for health professionals. Also, it is my hope that readers will recommend this book to various interdisciplinary health professionals who care for patients and residents. I'm convinced that no one discipline can solve the problem of falls by itself, but rather, it will take an interdisciplinary approach to be successful in preventing falls.

To the most important woman in my life:
my buddy and my soul mate, E.
The joy of your love
helps me grow younger and live longer

introduction

One of the most common and often critical problems faced by institutionally based health care providers is that of falls among older adults. Hospital falls represent a leading cause of adverse events, accounting for 25%–89% of all reported inpatient incidents.[1] To a large extent, this wide range is attributable to differences in various institutional policies (i.e., how falls are defined and reported) and the specific site or location of fall occurrence (e.g., rehabilitation, psychiatric, critical care, orthopedic, medical, surgical). For instance, in sub-acute or rehabilitation settings up to 46% of patients fall,[2] and in psychiatric hospitals, up to 36% of patients experience one or more falls.[3] In addition, more than 50% of falls in hospitals are not witnessed,[4] which is another factor responsible for inexact knowledge of fall frequencies.

Regardless of exactly how many people fall, people age 65 and older experience the majority of these falls. Studies that compare the age distribution of people with falls show that older people are overrepresented,[5,6] averaging about 1.5 falls per bed annually.[7] As many as 50% of these older inpatients fall repeatedly.[8] In the nursing facility, a setting to which older people are often admitted for safety reasons, falling is equally problematic. More than 50% of all nursing facility residents fall each year, and greater than 40% experience recurrent episodes.[9,10] The probability of falling, in both hospitals and nursing facilities, increases with advancing age; the highest incidence of falling occurs in the 80- to 89-year-old age group.[11,12] This high incidence is more a reflection of the increasing illness and frailty that accompanies aging than it is of old age itself. Falls, particularly repeated falls, are a major cause of physical and psychological trauma. Falls that occur repeatedly are likely to produce a cumulative adverse

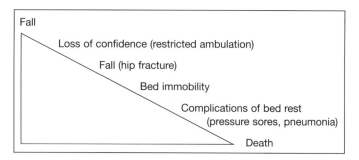

Figure I-1.   The downward-spiraling effects of falls.

effect on the individual's capacity for mobility, causing periods of immobility and, as an outcome of complications, premature death (see
Figure I-1).

In an effort to prevent falls, health care professionals have tried
to protect patients and residents by limiting their mobility, often resorting to the use of mechanical or chemical restraints. However,
mobility restrictions and restraint use have proven to be ineffective
in reducing falls and are associated with a host of negative outcomes
for older people. Moreover, federal and state governing bodies responsible for regulating hospitals and nursing facilities are focusing
their attention on the problem of mechanical and chemical restraints
and the methods employed to reduce them. In particular, they have
stated strongly that mechanical restraints have a very limited role
in the prevention of falls and are asking institutions to implement
restraint-reduction programs. A better understanding of the phenomenon of falls will help health care professionals to prevent falls
without resorting to traditional methods of restraint use.

Historically, the blame for falling has, for the most part, been
borne by the host, the person who falls. Popular mythology holds that
falls are attributable to either individual carelessness or the process
of aging. Falls are considered to be either a "normal" phenomenon of
aging—a manifestation of a general decline that is bound to occur—
or, in people with multiple disorders, one aspect of a "hopeless" state
in which one disorder after another leads inevitably to a negative con-
clusion. Many health care providers have dealt with falls and their adverse consequences for so long that they have become hardened; they

no longer identify them as problems with solutions, other than to restrict the individuals' mobility. Moreover, providers may be reluctant to consider the possibility of better solutions.

Contrary to popular myth, falls, to a large degree, rarely "just happen"—they are neither accidental nor random events—but are predictable occurrences, the outcome of a multitude of host-related and environmental factors that occur either alone or in conjunction with one another. Many of the factors that contribute to falls are potentially amenable to interventions. By minimizing or eliminating these risk factors, falls can be reduced or prevented altogether.

In order to implement preventive measures, health care providers must take the following steps. First, they must understand the conditions under which falls occur and the factors that are associated with fall risk. With an increased knowledge of why older people fall and what factors are associated with fall risk, providers will be able to more easily identify patients and residents at risk and explore appropriate solutions aimed at reducing fall risk. Many of the factors responsible for falls are quite easy to fix, particularly for someone with a practiced eye, a different perspective, and different expertise. The second step health care providers must take is to mount an organized approach to the clinical assessment of fall risk and falls and put in place intervention strategies for both.

Although hospitals and nursing facilities more or less differ in their goals, distribution and orientation of staff, population of individuals cared for, and environmental design principles (see Table I-1), the factors associated with falls as well as intervention strategies within each institution are similar in many respects. An apple-to-apple comparison between the two institutional settings may not always be possible—for instance, what works for hospitals with respect to preventing falls may not work for nursing facilities and vice versa—so when it becomes necessary to consider the specificity of each institution, it is noted and differences appropriate to each are set forth.

Falls are complex problems, often associated with a variety of causes. A great deal is known about older adults and falls; a wealth of information is available on their causes, and more important, on how to prevent falls. The challenge is how to take what is known and apply it. Although there is no "quick fix" for preventing falls, evidence suggests that an organized approach toward identifying patients and residents at risk for falling and targeting interventions

Table I-1. Characteristics of hospitals and nursing facilities

Characteristic	Hospitals	Nursing facilities
Goal	Diagnose and treat acute disease	Manage chronic disease
Population	Patients are medically unstable (i.e., are experiencing acute illness and/or exacerbations of chronic disease) Institutional stay is temporary	Residents are medically stable but require ongoing medical or personal assistance In general, institutional stay is long term
Staff	Acute care orientation Daily physician presence Higher nursing staff–patient ratio	Chronic care orientation Irregular physician presence Lower nursing staff–patient ratio
Environment	Designed to facilitate acute medical care services	Designed to accommodate residents' level of function

aimed at reducing risk is beneficial. To achieve this goal, health care professionals in hospitals and nursing facilities need to make a serious, long-term commitment to addressing the problem of falls as they apply to their individualized setting by developing clinical programs focused on preventing falls.

Content of the Book

The book is divided into two sections. Section One gives an overview and specific suggestions for helping the reader understand the underlying causes of falls and how to develop and maintain an effective falls management program. Chapter One examines the outcome of falls with respect to their consequences in patients and residents, their families, and the institution. Chapter Two reviews the multiple age-related physiological changes, pathological conditions, medications, and environmental and institutional factors associated with falls and fall risk. The clinical approach to the assessment of both falls and fall risk is examined in Chapter Three. Chapter Four explores a number of medical, rehabilitative, and environmental strategies that reduce fall risk. Common environmental causes of falling (e.g., lighting conditions, ground surfaces, furnishings) and their modifications are covered in Chapter Five. Chapter Six is devoted to a discussion of the issues surrounding mechanical and chemical restraints in the management of falls.

Section Two is divided into two parts. Part A provides guidelines, while Part B provides helpful photocopiable forms referenced throughout the book. Guidelines include a "best clinical practice" approach to the management of falls and fall risk in acute care hospitals and nursing facilities. Guidelines are also provided to help readers understand the structure and process of fall prevention and restraint-avoidance programs (i.e., what is needed and what has to happen in order to achieve success).

Forms include the comprehensive Performance-Oriented Environmental Mobility Screen (POEMS), as well as a restraint and nonrestraint assessment and care planning tool, a wheelchair problems and modifications checklist, and discharge teaching sheets that can be given to families when a patient leaves a facility to ensure the optimum safety of the individual at risk of falling at home.

ENDNOTES

1. Maciorowiski, L.F., Bruno, B., Dietrick-Gallagher, M., McNew, C., Sheppard-Hinkel, E., Wanich, C., & Regan, P. (1988). A review of the patient fall literature. *Journal of Nursing Quality Assurance*, *3*, 18–27.
2. Tutuarima, J., van der Meulen, J., de Haan, R., van Straten, A., & Limberg, M. (1997). Risk factors for falls of hospitalized stroke patients. *Stroke*, *28*, 297–301.
3. Tay, S.C., Quek, C., Pariyasami, S., Ong, B.S., Wee, B.M., Yeo, J., & Yeo, S. (2000). Fall incidence in a state psychiatric hospital in Singapore. *Journal of Psychosocial Nursing*, *38*, 11–16.
4. Nyberg, L., & Gustafson, Y. (1995). Patient falls in stroke rehabilitation: A challenge in rehabilitation strategies. *Stroke*, *26*, 838–842.
5. Goodwin, M.B., & Westbrook, J.I. (1993). An analysis of patient accidents in hospital. *Australian Clinical Review*, *13(3)*, 141–149.
6. Rigby, K., Clark, R., & Runciman, W. (1999). Adverse events in health care: Setting priorities based on economic evaluation. *Journal of Quality Clinical Practice*, *19*, 7–12.
7. Rubenstein, L.Z., Robbins, A.S., Schulman, B.L., Rosado, J., Osterweil, D., & Josephson, K.R. (1988). Falls and instability in the elderly. *Journal of the American Geriatrics Society*, *36*, 278–288.
8. Gaebler, S. (1993). Predicting which patient will fall . . . and fall again. *Journal of Advanced Nursing*, *18*, 1895–1902.

9. Nygaard, H. (1998). Falls and psychotropic drug consumption in long-term care residents: Is there an obvious association? *Gerontology, 44*, 46–50.

10. Kiely, D., Kiel, D., Burrows, A., & Lipsitz, L. (1998). Identifying nursing home residents at risk for falling. *Journal of American Geriatrics Society, 46*, 551–555.

11. Luukinen, H., Koski, L., Hiltunen, L., & Kivela, S.L. (1994). Incidence rate of falls in an aged population in northern Finland. *Journal of Clinical Epidemiology, 47*, 843–850.

12. Rubenstein, L.Z., Robbins, A.S., Josephson, K.R., Schulman, B.L., & Osterweil, D. (1990). The value of assessing falls in an elderly population: A randomized clinical trial. *Annals of Internal Medicine, 113*, 308–316.

understanding falls and falls management

chapter one

consequences of falls

Falls represent a major cause of death and disability in older people and pose a serious threat to their health and well being. The consequences of falls are not confined to older people. They place a burden on family members, make excessive demands on health care professionals, and strain the resources of institutions.

MORTALITY

Falls and their consequences are a leading cause of death in people 65 years old and older.[1] About 10,000 older adults die each year as a result of falls.[2, 3] The risk of dying from a fall increases as people age. Fall-related death rates among people 65 years old and older are 10–150 times higher than those in younger age groups. Of all deaths due to falls, 66% involve people age 75 or older; these individuals have a mortality rate eight times higher than that for people 65–74 years of age.[3] More than two thirds of injury-reported deaths after age 85 are related to falls.[4] Of those individuals admitted to the hospital after a fall, only about 50% will be alive 1 year later. Within the hospital setting, about 10% of older patients who have fallen die before discharge. In nursing facilities, approximately 1,800 fatal falls occur annually.[4] For people age 85 and older, it is estimated that one in every five falls results in death.[5] A clustering of falls (i.e., multiple falls occurring over a relatively short period of time) is associated with increased mortality.[6] (For the definition of this term and others used throughout this chapter, see the Terminology sidebar on page 4.)

Fall-related mortality appears to be the direct result of the fall (e.g., from injuries sustained) and current comorbidity (e.g., pneumo-

terminology

Clustering of falls	Multiple falling events occurring over a short period of time
Colles fracture	Distal forearm fracture (or fracture of the wrist)
Comorbidity	Presence of additional diseases or illnesses
Contraction (of joint)	Shortening or tightening of a muscle that causes decreased joint motion
Femoral neck	Head of the long bone of the thigh
Orthostatic hypotension	Lowered blood pressure that occurs on rising to an erect position
Osteoporosis	Decrease in bone strength
Protective reflex	Extension of the arms outward and/or a shift of the feet to maintain balance and avoid a fall
Pulmonary embolism	Blockage of pulmonary artery or one of its branches
Soft-tissue injury	Injury to nonbony tissues, for example, sprains and strains
Subdural hematoma	Accumulation of blood resulting from injury to the brain
Venous stasis	Blood trapped in an extremity (e.g., arm, leg) by compression of veins
Vestibular function	Mechanism within the inner ear involved in balance control

nia, heart failure, pulmonary disease). Older people have decreased body reserves or lower thresholds, and, once injured from a fall, they have a much higher likelihood of dying than do younger people. The use of mechanical restraints to guard against the risk of falls also has been implicated as a cause of death. Most commonly, with the restraint device in place, a person falls or climbs out of bed, slides off a chair, or slips downward in a raised hospital bed. He or she becomes entangled and suspended in the restraint—which is usually pressed tightly against the chest or throat—and dies from asphyxia.[7]

MORBIDITY

The consequences of falls are numerous, from physical injury to immobility, to psychosocial trauma, to a morbid fear of falling again.

Physical Injury

Half of all hospitalizations resulting from injurious falls are experienced by people older than age 65, and people hospitalized for fall-related trauma are discharged to nursing facilities more often than are individuals without falls. Within the institutional setting, an estimated 16% of falls occurring to older people result in physical injury; approximately 4% result in fractures, and approximately 12% result in other serious injuries such as head injuries, soft-tissue injuries, musculoskeletal sprains, and lacerations.[5] The most common fractures are those of the distal forearm and hip. Distal forearm, or *Colles* fractures, occur when an older person loses balance and attempts to break a fall in progress by extending the arms outward. After age 70, there is a decrease in the incidence of forearm fractures, at which time there is a steep increase in the incidence of hip fractures and head injuries. An older person's decreased ability to exhibit the protective reflex is usually given as the cause of the decline in distal forearm fractures.

Some hypothesize that a decline in the protective reflex may be attributed to age-related changes in central nervous system function (e.g., decreased reaction and response times), concomitant diseases (e.g., stroke, Parkinson's disease, arthritis), and certain drugs (e.g., psychotropics, hypnotics).[8] Consequently, older people who fall are at great risk for head trauma, spinal cord trauma, and hip fracture.

Falls are a leading cause of head injury in older people. Aside from bruises and lacerations, subdural hematomas are the most significant head injuries. They tend to occur more frequently than other injuries because of certain age-related changes in the older brain such as decreased cerebral reserve. As a result, older people are less able than younger people to withstand even minor trauma such as might occur from bumping into a wall, a bed side rail, or a headboard. Any time a person exhibits mental confusion following a fall, a neurological evaluation should be conducted to rule out a subdural hematoma. Any lingering subdural hematoma that has not healed within a relatively short period of time can lead to permanent cognitive dysfunction. Approximately 2.9% of falls result in hip fracture.[9] Although the incidence of hip fractures is low, the subsequent mortality and morbidity is substantial. Of all hip fracture patients, 4% die in the hospital,[10] and within 1 year after their injury, up to 23% are dead;[11] people 75 years old and older have the highest mortality rates.[1] A high incidence of coexisting chronic diseases in people with hip fracture contributes to this increased mortality rate. After a hip fracture, many older people never regain their premorbid level of ambulation. Approximately 60% of people have decreased mobility; another 25% become functionally dependent in walking and require mechanical assistance (e.g., the use of a cane or walker) or the assistance of another person.[1] Of all hip fracture survivors, 14% remain in the nursing facility 1 year after injury.[12]

The risk of sustaining a hip fracture from a fall is dependent on a number of interacting factors, including the height of the fall and impact surface, protective reflexes, "shock absorbers," and bone strength.

Height of the Fall and Impact Surface   In order to build sufficient momentum to produce injury (e.g., bone fracture), an individual must fall a considerable distance. For example, an unexpected fall from a standing height (e.g., from a slip, from a loss of consciousness) or a fall from an elevated bed height (e.g., over bed side rails) is more likely to result in injury because of the increased force of impact than a fall from a relatively low height, such as from a chair or toilet. Falls on hard, nonabsorptive floor surfaces such as linoleum tile, concrete, and wood are more likely to result in injury than falls onto absorptive surfaces such as carpeting.

Protective Reflexes   The onset of a fall elicits several protective reflexes, including extending the arms outward and initiating quick shifting movements of the feet in order to regain balance. Both may avert a fall or minimize the force of impact. Conversely, a loss of protective reflexes stemming from neuromuscular dysfunction that affects the extremities or from sedation induced by medication may increase the impact of falling and the risk of injury.

"Shock Absorbers" The presence of increased fat and muscle bulk surrounding vulnerable areas, such as the hip, is capable of absorbing the impact of a fall, decreasing the risk of fracture. Fractures are more likely to occur in people whose muscles have atrophied or who have a decreased amount of fat padding (i.e., thin people).

Bone Strength A loss of bone strength attributable to osteoporosis at the femoral neck may result in fractures. These fractures may be either "spontaneous" hip fractures that occur during weight-bearing episodes or fractures that occur even with minimal ground impact against the bone. Bone loss is a particular problem in older women: By age 80, women may have lost up to 50% of their bone strength, compared with 15% in men.

Immobility In the absence of physical injury, falls are often associated with a restriction of activities—either self- or staff-imposed—and immobility. As a consequence, people are at risk for a host of morbid complications that increase with the duration of immobility (Table 1-1). In turn, any concomitant loss of functional status places individuals at additional risk for falls (Figure 1-1).

Psychosocial Trauma

Falls, particularly those that recur, are associated with a number of traumatic psychosocial consequences. Threats of impending falls can alter self-image and create feelings of increasing frailty and incompetence. Often, people experience increased anxiety during the performance of the activities of daily living (ADLs; e.g., getting out of bed, transferring from the toilet) because they are uncertain as to whether the ADLs can be accomplished safely. Such people become increasingly apprehensive, and their sense of vulnerability to falling and self-injury is heightened. These individuals may become depressed, especially if their mobility or freedom to move about independently is diminished and they become functionally dependent on staff for assistance. Any limitations in mobility have broad lifestyle implications for these older adults. For example, they may remain in their rooms or sit alone in the unit, which decreases their sociability and participation in leisure activities. Often, compromised mobility that becomes permanent necessitates individuals being placed in long-term care facilities. Falls and immobility account for up to one

Table 1-1.   Physiological and psychological consequences of immobility

System	Consequences
Musculoskeletal	Joint contractions, causing decreased range of motion
	Muscle weakness/atrophy
	Osteoporosis
Integumentary	Pressure sores
Respiratory	Pneumonia, causing decreased ventilation
	Pulmonary embolism
Cardiovascular	Orthostatic hypotension
	Venous stasis
Urinary	Urinary infections
	Incontinence
Gastrointestinal	Constipation
Neurological	Vestibular dysfunction/loss of balance
Psychological	Social isolation
	Decreased self-image
	Depression
	Anxiety
	Confusion

third of all admissions to nursing facilities,[13] thus constituting one of the leading causes of nursing facility placement.

Patients and residents with falls may voice a number of other worries or fears, which include the following:

- Being belted or restrained, experiencing a loss of autonomy
- Having their relatives informed of the episode, which may cause further embarrassment for the patient or resident
- Being transferred to "dependent" units for their care, thus experiencing a loss of independence
- Fearing that nursing staff will not be available or come to their aid in time to prevent another fall from taking place
- Being forced to use a cane or walker, thus losing self-esteem
- Becoming a burden to family and staff members
- Dreading another injury, that the next fall will result in a hip fracture

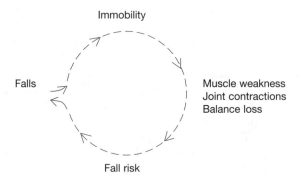

Immobility

Falls

Muscle weakness
Joint contractions
Balance loss

Fall risk

Figure 1-1. Falls that are associated with immobility and subsequent functional decline can increase the risk of additional falls.

Fear of Falling

Falls can lead to patients or residents losing confidence in their ability to function because of a fear of falling. Conservative estimates indicate that up to 50% of people who fall avoid ADLs because they fear additional falls and injury.[14] Such fear may be protective or it may be harmful. To a certain degree, it may be protective if it motivates people to avoid activities to which they are no longer equal, to recognize their limitations, and to become more cautious. However, a fear of falling also can be detrimental, adversely affecting mobility and independence. As a response to their fear, some individuals alter their walking patterns; typically, their steps become hesitant and irregular.

Ambulation is accompanied by a great deal of anxiety and often is accomplished by the person clutching or grabbing onto furnishings for support, a strategy that may increase the risk of falls. Subsequently, many people experience multiple near-falls, which can heighten their fear of falling and may lead to a curtailment of all physical activity. Devices that assist in safe mobility are often rejected because many older people are reluctant to project an image of frailty and thus endure social rejection from their peers, or they may feel that their cane or walker provides insufficient support. Other people who are fearful of falling may eventually become chairbound or bedridden, reluctant to attempt independent activities, and in need of human assistance to accomplish ADLs. Many patients and residents in this category develop a fear of being dropped by staff members during transfer activities and may be hesitant to leave their beds or chairs. Fear of falling may lead to a number of morbid outcomes. Older hospital patients may delay or eventually avoid discharge to the community, particularly if they live alone. Stalling can affect these patients adversely because many times it ultimately leads to placement in a nursing facility. Similarly, many nursing facility residents with a fear of falling become socially isolated and functionally dependent. Thus, the risk of complications associated with immobility increases.

FAMILY CONCERNS

Family members of people with falls in hospitals and nursing facilities also experience the consequences of falls. They may feel guilty about the fall, blaming themselves for not "being there" to prevent the event, or they may blame the nursing staff for allowing the fall to happen, sometimes even accusing the staff of neglect. Concerned for the safety of their relative, family members may insist on restricting activities and may inquire about the use of mechanical restraints and bed side rails to safeguard the patient or resident. These restrictions are especially likely to occur if the older person experiences multiple falls or a fall that results in injury. Although many family members become dismayed at the sight of restraints, they reluctantly accept their use for safety reasons. Other families, however, may insist on restraint removal, even if it places their loved ones at risk for falls. Most families do not seek a guarantee that no harm will come to their relative, but rather, assurance that the staff will assess the problem or the risk for subsequent falls and take appropriate measures to guard against falls. When alternatives to the use of mechanical restraints are discussed with family members, they often feel comfortable with the concept of reducing or eliminating restraints.

In the hospital setting, many families question staff about whether their loved ones can safely return home, particularly if they live alone. Families seek alternatives such as altered living arrangements (e.g., moving the relative with falls in with them) or placement in a group home or assisted living facility. If these options are not feasible, families may resort to nursing facility placement.

INSTITUTIONAL EFFECTS

The consequences of falls are challenging for institutions as well as families and the individuals themselves. The complications include increased health care costs and effects on staff.

Health Care Costs

Falls and their complications often result in increased costs from potential liability risks as well as health care needs. The institution and its employees are responsible for the safety of their patients or residents for the length of their stay in the institution and may be held responsible if older adults fall and sustain injuries. Thus, both institution and staff are at risk for legal liability and increased costs associated with legal fees and settlement awards. Falls are the largest category of incident reports submitted to risk management for review because of potential liability.[15] The risk of legal action is highest in patients and residents whose falls are associated with serious injury, such as a fracture. Family members, rather than the patients and residents themselves, are likely to file a complaint against the institution, perhaps partly because of guilt about their relative's poor outcome.

Falls and injuries generate other expenses as well, including

- *Labor costs:* nursing, physician, and rehabilitative services accrued as a result of the time spent evaluating fall events, completing documentation (e.g., filling out occurrence reports, charting), providing postfall care (e.g., treating injury and immobility complications, restorative care), and monitoring patients and residents at fall risk (e.g., hourly nursing rounds, in-room sitters)
- *Equipment costs:* mobility devices (e.g., canes, walkers, wheelchairs), bed rails, bed alarm systems, and durable medical equipment (e.g., grab bars, toileting devices, restraints, restraint-alternative devices)

- *Utilization costs:* prolonged hospitalization (e.g., increased length of stay, increased bed-days) and permanent placement, in the case of nursing facilities; recurrent falls and their complications are common causes of rehospitalization and readmission to nursing facilities

Many times, institutions must bear the brunt of these expenses. Hospital reimbursement systems may not pay for services required or extended days due to complications that stem from falls and injuries. In nursing facilities with reimbursement capitation, the necessary care that results from fall-related complications may exceed coverage. In general, hospitals and nursing facilities that hold capitation contracts with managed care organizations are responsible for any expenses accumulated, and managed care plans that enroll residents of nursing facilities are responsible for covering fall-related costs.

Effects on Staff

Nursing staff caring for patients and residents with recurrent falls may find the responsibility of constantly deciding between the individuals' desire for autonomy and the families' requests for safety and protection against the risk of falls emotionally demanding. Staff easily can become disheartened when patients and residents continue to fall, despite all their attempts to prevent falls. Often, staff may experience stress, guilt, and self-doubt about their ability to deliver safe care.

ENDNOTES

1. Davis, A.E. (1995). Hip fractures in the elderly: Surveillance methods and injury control. *Journal of Nursing Trauma, 2*(1), 15–21.
2. Centers for Disease Control and Prevention. (1995). *Injury mortality, 1986–1992.* Atlanta: Author.
3. Centers for Disease Control and Prevention. (1996). *National summary of injury mortality data, 1988–1994.* Atlanta: Author.
4. Baker, S.P., O'Neill, B., Ginsburg, M.J., & Guohua, L. (1992). *The injury fact book (2nd ed.).* New York: Oxford University Press.
5. Rubenstein, L.Z., Josephson, K.P., & Osterweil, D. (1996). Falls and fall prevention in the nursing home. *Clinics in Geriatric Medicine, 12*(4), 881–902.

6. Wolinsky, F.D., Johnson, R.J., & Fitzgerald, J.F. (1992). Falling, health status, and use of health services by older adults. *Medical Care, 30,* 587–597.
7. Miles, S.H., & Irvine, P.I. (1992). Deaths caused by physical restraints. *Gerontologist, 32,* 762–766.
8. Melton, L.J., Chao, E.Y.S., & Lane, J. (1988). Biomechanical aspects of fractures. In B.L. Briggs & L.J. Melton (Eds.), *Osteoporosis: Etiology, diagnosis, and management (pp. 111–131).* New York: Raven Press.
9. Sattin, R.W. (1992). Falls among older persons: A public health perspective. *Annual Review of Public Health, 13,* 489–508.
10. U.S. Department of Health and Human Services, Public Health Service, National Center for Health Statistics. (1992). *Unpublished data from the 1988 and 1991 National Hospital Discharge Survey.* Washington, DC: Author.
11. Fisher, E.S., Baron, J., Malenka, D.I., Barrett, J.A., Kniffin, W.D., Whaley, F.S., & Bubolz, T.A. (1991). Hip fracture mortality in New England. *Epidemiology, 2(2),* 116–122.
12. Kennedy, E.M. (1994). *Hip fracture outcomes in people age fifty and over— Background paper.* OTA-BP-H-120. Washington, DC: U.S. Government Printing Office.
13. Tinetti, M.E., & Speechley, M. (1989). Prevention of falls among the elderly. *New England Journal of Medicine, 320,* 1055–1059.
14. Franzoni, S., Ronzzini, R., Boffelli, S., Frisoni, E.B., & Trabucchi, M. (1994). Fear of falling in nursing home patients. *Gerontology, 40,* 38–44.
15. Quinlan, W.C. (1994). The liability risk of patients who fall. *Journal of Healthcare Risk Management, 14,* 29–33.

causes of falling
and fall risk

A fall can be defined as any event in which a person inadvertently or intentionally comes to rest on the ground or another low level such as a chair, toilet, or bed. As an initial step in designing any planned intervention to reduce falls, it is essential to know why falls occur and under what circumstances they take place. The risk of falling occurs when an individual engages in an activity that results in a loss of balance, a displacement of the body beyond its base of support. Loss of balance may occur while carrying out everyday activities such as walking; transferring on or off chairs, wheelchairs, beds, and toilets; and reaching up or bending to retrieve or place objects. A fall is likely to follow an episode of balance loss if the neuromuscular systems responsible for balance stability fail to recognize and correct the displacement of the body in time to avert a fall.

Falls in older people are often precipitated by a number of factors. These factors encompass intrinsic factors (e.g., age-related physiological changes, disease states, medications) as well as extrinsic factors (e.g., hazardous environmental conditions, faulty devices, footwear). In addition, several situational circumstances, such as length of stay in institutional settings, time of day when falls take place, and staff characteristics, influence the occurrence of falls.

Falling should be viewed as a nonspecific sign or symptom representative of an underlying problem that can be attributed to either intrinsic or extrinsic factors. In the past, falls have been assigned to a single cause and ascribed either to a medical event or "accidental" environmental encounter. As researchers are beginning to understand, in general, falls in older people are not the result of a single

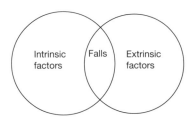

Figure 2-1. Falls are caused by the interaction of intrinsic and extrinsic factors.

intrinsic or extrinsic factor occurring in isolation; rather, falls are complex events caused by a combination of both factors (Figure 2-1). However, for ease of understanding the etiology, or causes, of falls, it is useful to divide falls into strict intrinsic and extrinsic categories.

INTRINSIC FACTORS

A number of intrinsic factors play an important role in fall causation. These factors consist of age-related changes (e.g., changes in vision, changes in balance, changes in gait, changes in the musculoskeletal system, changes in the cardiovascular system), pathological conditions (e.g., acute diseases, chronic diseases), and medications.

Age-Related Changes

Mobility, the ability to maintain upright posture and to ambulate and transfer effectively, depends on the operation and integrity of many systems, primarily the visual, neurological, musculoskeletal, and cardiovascular systems. With advancing age, these systems decline gradually in function; they affect gait and balance and influence the risk of falling.

Changes in Vision The ability of the eyes to adjust to varying levels of light and darkness diminishes as people age. As a result, the eyes of older people require more time to adjust to changes in environmental lighting. Dark adaptation is especially affected by aging and may compromise a person's visual capacity, particularly under conditions of low illumination (e.g., when walking about or toileting during nighttime hours). When moving from a dimly lit room into bright lighting and vice versa, people often experience temporary blindness until the eyes adjust to the dramatic change in illumination.

A greater sensitivity of the aging eye to glare can lead to visual dysfunction. Common sources of glare include sunlight shining through windows and reflecting off waxed floors or glossy tabletops and bright light from unshielded light and fluorescent bulbs directed toward the eye. Glare from floor surfaces is particularly troublesome because it can mask potential ground surface hazards. Also, glare can create visual distortions in older people that may result in their perceiving floor surfaces as excessively slippery. As a consequence, individuals sometimes alter their gait to compensate. They walk slower and more flat-footed and use a wider base of support, a pattern reminiscent of that which people adopt to walk on ice. However, this gait change may not be safe and can lead to unsteadiness and falls. At other times, people cope with the glare emanating from floors by avoiding the surface altogether. Some view excessive floor glare, especially if it restricts an individual's mobility, as a passive form of restraint (for a definition of glare and other terms, see the Terminology sidebar on pages 18–20).

Restriction of a person's visual field leads to an inability to see objects in the pathway that lies outside the person's view, increasing the likelihood of slips and trips. A loss of visual acuity and contrast sensitivity can make the perception of objects in the environment more difficult. In particular, the detection of low-contrast objects can lead to unsafe ambulation and transferring activity. If not visualized clearly, objects such as extended chair and table legs, door thresholds, and carpet edges can cause people to trip. Furnishing surfaces (e.g., chair and toilet seats, bed mattress edges) that are not visually distinguishable can interfere with the achievement of proper stable seating positions, which increases the likelihood of falls while transferring. The loss of visual acuity and contrast sensitivity or decreased functional vision is more evident under conditions of low illumination (e.g., walking to the bathroom at night).

A decline in depth perception can cause the visual detection of certain ground surfaces (e.g., patterned or checkered linoleum, carpet designs) to appear to be elevations or depressions on the ground, surfaces that older people prefer to step around or avoid walking on entirely. In addition, a loss of depth perception makes it difficult to perceive objects that lie in areas of shadows, low illumination, or excessive brightness.

terminology

Agnosia	Neurological disorder that leads to disturbances in the recognition or perception of familiar sensory information
Apraxia	Loss of the ability to execute previously learned motor skills
Ataxia	Impairment of coordination of muscular activity
Cardiac arrhythmia	Any deviation from the normal pace of the heart
Cardio-acceleration	An increase in the pulse rate
Cervical spondylosis	Breakdown of cervical vertebrae
Chronic obstructive pulmonary disease	General term for disease involving airway obstruction (e.g., chronic bronchitis, emphysema, asthma)
Congestive heart failure	Chronic inability of the heart to maintain an adequate output of blood, resulting in an inadequate blood supply to the body
Contrast sensitivity	The ability to perceive spatial detail and object contrast
Dark adaptation	The ability of the eyes to adjust to low levels of illumination
Dorsiflexion	Bending or flexing
Dysarthria	Difficulty in articulating single sounds in speech
Dysphasia	Disturbance in speech evidenced by lack of coordination and failure to express words in proper order
Electrolyte disorders	Disorder in compounds that play an essential role in function of the body
Extracellular volume regulation	Homeostatic mechanisms that regulate against volume depletion
Extrinsic	External to the system

Gait cycle	The manner of progression in walking or style of walking
Glare	A dazzling effect associated with a source of intense illumination
Hemianopsia	Blindness in half of the visual field
Hemiplegia	Paralysis involving one side of the body, generally an arm or leg
Hypotension	Low blood pressure
Hypovolemia	Low fluid states in the body
Intrinsic	Integral to the system
Kyphosis	Dorsal curvature of the spine in the thoracic area (i.e., hunchback)
Low-contrast objects	Objects whose color is similar or indistinguishable from the immediate background
Macular degeneration	Eye condition, probably hereditary, causing diminished central vision
Marker	Early sign or indication of a corollary or subsequent event/disease
Nocturia	Excessive nighttime urination
Orthostatic hypotension	Lowered blood pressure that occurs on rising to an erect position
Osteomalacia	Softening of the bones
Paresis	Slight or incomplete paralysis; weakness
Peripheral neuropathy	Disease of the nerves
Polypharmacy	Use of multiple medications
Prodromal falls	Falling events that precede an episode of illness
Proprioception	Sense providing the body with kinesthetic information on the immediate environment, which enables the body to orient itself in space without visual clues; proprioception emerges from muscles, tendons, and joint receptors

(continued)

terminology   *(continued)*

Propulsion	An uncontrolled forward motion
Proximal muscles	Muscles of the thighs, upper arms, and shoulders
Retropulsion	Loss of balance in a backward direction
Step length	The distance the foot travels during the swing phase
Steppage height	The level of ground clearance by the foot during the swing phase
Syncope	Fainting; temporary unconsciousness
Synergistic effects of medications	Accumulated effects of multiple medications
Vasomotor instability	Affecting the caliber of blood vessels—leads to inconsistent blood flow
Vestibular input	Signals that convey linear (angular) acceleration of the head; contributes to balance maintenance
Vestibular receptors	The semicircular canals and otolith organs located in the ear

Changes in Balance   The body's ability to maintain balance depends on the central nervous and musculoskeletal systems, requiring adequate vision, proprioceptive feedback, vestibular input, muscle strength, and joint flexibility to detect and correct balance displacement. Combined, these systems culminate in postural sway, a process of antero-posterior and lateral motion of the standing or seated body that controls stability and protects against the forces of gravity (i.e., loss of balance and falls).

Balance is achieved by the body's continual positioning of its center of gravity over a base of support: the feet, when standing (Figure 2-2), and the buttocks, when sitting (Figure 2-3). When an individual performs an activity such as walking or transferring, his or her center of gravity extends beyond the base of support and stretches beyond the limits of stability (Figure 2-4). The resulting imbalance is detected by the visual, vestibular, and proprioceptive components of the central nervous system, which sends signals to stretch receptors located in the joints and muscles of the legs. This signaling initiates a set of coordinated protective movements (e.g., a forward or backward shifting of the feet while standing or walking, a widening of the feet while seated or transferring) that pulls the body's center of gravity into alignment with its base of support.

As people age, the capabilities of the proprioceptive system decline and, as a consequence, postural sway increases. Vision can augment proprioceptive feedback or counteract its loss. To compensate for poor balance, many individuals ambulate by looking down to view the correct placement of their feet; to ensure proper transferring, they constantly view the surface on which they sit. Vision is a mainstay of balance. The eyes provide the body with information on the placement of and distance from objects in the environment, the type of surface on which movement will take place, the position of the body, and the intensity of effort or degree of difficulty of the required movement. Vision also provides the information the person needs to think ahead of time and to gauge the timing and control of movement. The more difficult the activity or the greater the

Figure 2-2. The center of gravity in relationship to the base of support when standing.

precision and speed needed to accomplish the movement, the greater the importance of vision. When visual input is diminished by age-related changes, balance becomes difficult to maintain. This concept is demonstrated when an older person stands with his or her eyes closed or walks into a dark room; in both cases, balance is unsteady.

Figure 2-3. The center of gravity in relationship to the base of support when seated.

The vestibular system works in conjunction with the visual and proprioceptive systems to achieve balance—it helps to maintain stable visual perception and body orientation as a person moves about the environment. During periods of displacement of balance,

Figure 2-4. The center of gravity in relationship to the base of support during (left) ambulation and (right) transfers.

the vestibular receptors detect movement and prompt antigravity extensor muscles to execute compensatory head, trunk, and limb movements, which serve to oppose postural sway. In other words, the system located in the inner ear that regulates balance senses that the body has been placed out of balance and signals the neuromuscular system to activate one or more movements to ensure that a fall does not take place. This body-orienting response, known as the righting reflex, diminishes with age. Consequently, when an older person slips or trips or loses balance while transferring, his or her chance of regaining stability and avoiding a fall declines.

Usually, some redundancy occurs in the sensory information necessary to maintain balance, and the failure of one source of input such as vision can be counteracted with feedback from intact proprioceptive and vestibular systems. However, deprivation in more than one system is likely to lower the balance threshold and increase fall risk. This risk becomes evident when older people who have fallen are compared with older people who have not fallen. Older people who fall have greater postural sway or unsteadiness than individuals without falls, and people with multiple falls demonstrate appreciably more sway or unsteady balance than those with single falls.[1]

Changes in Gait   The gait cycle consists of two phases: stance and swing. The stance phase occurs when one leg is in con-

Figure 2-5. (A) The stance phase and (B) the swing phase of the gait cycle.

tact with the ground, and the swing phase occurs when the other leg is advanced forward to take the next step (Figure 2-5). Ambulation is accomplished via a series of reciprocal leg movements that alternate between stance and swing—pushing off on the leg in stance phase while swinging the other leg forward. To allow for adequate ground clearance during the swing phase, the leg is flexed at the knee and dorsiflexed at the foot (Figure 2-6). When the heel of the swing leg strikes the ground, the return to the stance phase, the knee is extended and the foot is plantar flexed to provide support to the body (Figure 2-7).

Figure 2-7. Ground support during a return to the stance phase is accomplished by (A) knee extension and (B) ankle plantar flexion.

Figure 2-6. Ground clearance during the swing phase is accomplished by (A) knee flexion and (B) ankle dorsiflexion.

Figure 2-8. The gait of (A) an older person is compared with that of (B) a younger person, demonstrating a decrease in step length and steppage height.

As compared with younger people, older individuals experience a number of changes in the gait cycle. The speed of walking, step length, and steppage height declines (Figure 2-8). Changes in gait are also specific to each gender, although they are not well understood. Women tend to develop a narrow standing and walking base, often take small steps, and exhibit a pelvic waddle during ambulation. The pelvic waddle has been attributed, in part, to a loss of muscular control in the lower extremities. Conversely, older men tend to adopt a wide standing and walking base and assume a more shuffling type of gait.

Whether age-related changes in gait are compensatory and serve to maintain balance or are hazardous, and thus influence fall risk, remains speculative. Alterations in gait, however, are more evident in people with a history of falls and this influences fall susceptibility to a certain degree. When the swing phase is interrupted (Figure 2-9), either the foot fails to adequately clear the ground or it encounters an irregularity on the surface of the floor such as curled-up carpeting or a raised tile edge, which results in tripping. When a

Figure 2-9. The movement of the right foot is interrupted during the swing phase. A trip and fall forward occurs as a result.

Figure 2-10. The movement of the right foot during a return to the stance phase encounters a surface of low frictional resistance. A slip and fall backward occurs as a result.

bare foot or shoe bottom either encounters a surface of low frictional resistance (e.g., wet or highly polished floor surface) or approaches the ground with a change in stride length during a return to the stance phase, a slip can occur (Figure 2-10). Whether a trip or slip results in a fall depends on the ability of the individual to initiate and execute maneuvers that correct his or her balance.

Changes in the Musculoskeletal System   The capacity to maintain balance while walking and transferring, and thus accomplish these activities safely, is affected by a number of age-related changes in the musculoskeletal system. Such changes include muscle atrophy, calcification of tendons and ligaments, and increased curvature of the spine due to osteoporosis, which results in kyphosis. In response, older people develop a stooped posture (Figure 2-11) and have difficulty extending their hips and knees fully when walking, which can affect their ability to maintain stability and to correct any displacements of balance that may occur. A severe forward-leaning posture may alter the body's balance threshold: The center of gravity is shifted forward, past the base of support (i.e., the critical point of stability), making it more difficult for older people to thrust the foot forward quickly enough to preserve balance. Poor ankle muscle strength complicates the execution, and older people find it difficult to adjust their center of gravity in line with the base of support rapidly enough to prevent a fall. In fact, with age, general muscular strength declines, particularly in the proximal muscles.

The deterioration of articular cartilage in the hips and knees becomes prominent in older adults. In concert, these changes can impair transfer activity (e.g., sitting down and rising from chairs, toilets, and beds). An inability to flex the knees and hips sufficiently and the loss of lower extremity strength may impair the capacity of the legs to exert maximum push or force during the attempt to transfer. Similarly, a decrease in shoulder and upper extremity flexibility and strength may cause the body to fail to provide optimal upper extremity leverage during transfers.

Figure 2-11. Age-related musculoskeletal changes can lead to a stooped posture.

Changes in the Cardiovascular System

Aging is associated with several physiological changes that impair homeostasis or regulation of blood pressure, which can predispose older adults to falls. The baroreceptor reflex, which consists of stretch receptors located in large arteries, is sensitive to sudden changes in blood pressure and serves as a regulatory mechanism that helps to maintain sufficient blood flow to the brain. This reflex occurs despite changes in posture, such as suddenly standing up after remaining seated or in a prone position for some time. As people age, they experience a progressive decline in baroreflex stimulation, which is due to arteriosclerosis. This arterial hardening may cause transient episodes of hypotension, which becomes evident in the presence of hypotensive stimuli such as hypovolemia (e.g., dehydration, blood loss) or medication side effects. As such, the aged heart is less able than a younger heart to cardioaccelerate to compensate for any hypotensive effects. Also, older people have impaired extracellular volume regulation and, as a result, sodium conservation declines. Diminished sodium conservation can lead to sodium imbalance and dehydration, which can influence blood pressure regulation and subsequently lead to hypotension.

Pathological Conditions

Diseases and their associated impairments, superimposed on age-related physiological changes, play a more decisive role in falls than do physiological changes occurring by themselves. Older people possess considerable reserve capacity beyond what may be needed for ordinary mobility tasks. Therefore, aging per se and age-related physiological changes are less likely to cause falls in the absence of associated disease. Often, falls are markers for an underlying acute disease or diseases. Indeed, evidence indicates that, in general, people with repeated falls have more medical comorbidity than do individuals without falls.[2]

Acute Diseases A falling event may be the initial sign or an early indication of an underlying acute illness, representing the onset of new diseases or an unstable existing disease, as in the following case example:

B.R. is an 89-year-old man with severe Parkinson's disease who experienced five falls during a 2-week period. The falls were ascribed to poor mobility resulting from his neurological disease. Subsequent investigation, however, revealed the presence of a gastrointestinal bleed (i.e., blood in the stool with anemia), which was generated by a stomach ulcer. After treatment of the ulcer, his falls ceased.

Falling episodes that precede an episode of illness are referred to as prodromal falls. Illnesses most often identified as causative of falls are those present at the time of the fall that interfere with postural stability; such illnesses include syncope, hypotension, cardiac arrhythmias, electrolyte disorders, seizures, stroke, febrile conditions (e.g., urinary tract infections, pneumonia), and acute exacerbations of underlying chronic diseases (e.g., congestive heart failure, chronic obstructive pulmonary disease, kidney failure). Approximately 10% of falls in older people are attributed to acute illness.

Chronic Diseases Frequently, a fall heralds a deterioration in health that is attributable to a chronic disease. Disease processes that predispose to falls include any persistent physical condition that interferes with mobility (e.g., the ability to walk about the environment; safe transfer on and off chairs, beds, and toilets). The most common disease processes originate in the visual, neurological, and musculoskeletal systems. Degenerative cognitive disorders compound the effects of falls and create a high risk for them.

Visual Disorders Diseases of the eye such as cataracts, macular degeneration, glaucoma, and hemianopsia interfere with visual fields and decrease visual perception, visual acuity, and dark adaptation. Cataracts result in an overall blurring of vision, causing images to appear hazy or cloudy, and cause increased sensitivity to glare. Macular degeneration affects only central vision; peripheral vision remains intact. Glaucoma results in the loss of peripheral vision, and hemianopsia causes loss of vision in half of the visual field. When combined with poor illumination, visual disorders can result in poor recognition of environmental ground hazards and predispose individuals to trips and slips. Visual impairment interfering with safe mobility is especially a problem during nighttime hours.

Neurological Disorders Dementia, especially of the Alzheimer's type, is associated with neurological disorders: ataxia, proprioceptive loss, apraxia, visuospatial dysfunction in object recognition, and agnosia. These changes lead to misinterpretation of environmental conditions, resulting in trips and slips, balance loss, and a reduced ability to correct imbalance and falls.

Neuropathy—the result of conditions such as diabetes mellitus, vitamin B_{12} deficiency, and cervical spondylosis—is associated with lower extremity weakness and altered proprioception, which can lead to poor balance and abnormal gait. Lower extremity hemiplegia or paresis resulting from stroke can result in a narrow, unstable standing and walking base of support, which is maintained typically on the unaffected foot, and increases the risk of loss of balance. A decrease in ankle dorsiflexion of the affected limb results in a diminished ability to initiate quick postural responses, and reduced foot–ground clearance during ambulation precipitates tripping. Parkinsonism affects postural control; it institutes a loss of autonomic postural reflexes, propulsion, retropulsion, and certain gait changes (e.g., short-stepping and shuffling, barely clearing the ground; poor initiation; freezing or sudden halting of gait) that can lead to a displaced center of gravity, loss of balance, and fall risk.

Musculoskeletal Disorders Proximal muscle weakness, concomitant with conditions such as thyroid disease, polymyalgia rheumatica, osteomalacia, or deconditioning, can lead to unstable, waddling gaits and problems with transferring. Osteoarthritis of the knees and hips with limited joint flexibility may result in similar problems. Disorders of the foot (e.g., toe deformities, calluses, bunions) lead to mechanical problems during ambulation and to unsteady gaits.

Cognitive Disorders   Altered thought processes resulting from dementia or depression are associated with falls. Older adults may misperceive environmental dangers, err in judgment, or fail to discriminate between safe and dangerous environmental conditions or activities. Consequently, they may place themselves in hazardous situations and take chances that people who are cognitively intact would avoid. Individuals with dementia who wander, especially those with mobility problems, can be at particular risk, and they may lack the ability to communicate their needs. Conversely, despite their functional frailty, some people who are cognitively intact insist on maintaining a risky level of autonomy, particularly if they are accustomed to being active and independent. Their stubbornness can increase the risk of falls.

Language Disorders   Impaired communication attributable to conditions such as dysarthria and dysphagia may seriously compromise an older adult's safety. An inability to make one's wishes known (e.g., needing help with bed transfers, wanting to walk to the bathroom) or an inability to understand safety risks causes individuals to attempt activities when they may be inadvisable or risky. In addition, any frustration or anxiety resulting from a failure to communicate can increase the risk of falls. Avoiding a fall is likely not the primary concern of people who are frustrated or anxious. Rather, they become consumed emotionally by an immediate problem, such as toileting. As a result, individuals may be less alert to surrounding environmental hazards.

The management of patients and residents with communication deficits consists of identifying the language problems and any specific precautions needed to ensure their safety. In general, older adults need to be informed about hazardous activities and environmental conditions, as well as about ways to call for help when it is needed, despite the difficulty in communicating. The use of pictures, pantomime, notebooks, communication boards, and cards that have pictures of familiar objects should be encouraged. A speech-language pathologist can help to identify other communication-enhancing techniques.

Medications

Physiologic responses to medications change as people age.[3–5] A number of pharmacokinetic and pharmacodynamic changes take place, affecting how the body handles a drug, as well as the specific action of the drug on the body. Major pharmacokinetic alterations in the distribution, metabolism, and excretion of medications occur with aging. An increase in total body fat and decrease in lean muscle mass cause alterations in lipophilic, or fat-soluble, medications. For example, benzodiazepines and psychotropic medications delay clearance from the body and prolong the half-life of drugs. A decrease in total body water and albumin levels may lead to high serum levels of medications or accumulation of water-soluble and protein-binding drugs. The capacity of the liver to metabolize medications is also impaired, the effect being acute with benzodiazepines. A reduction in hepatic blood flow can decrease the clearance of drugs traveling through the liver, thus prolonging their half-lives. Psychotropics appear to be affected the most by the aging metabolism. A reduction in renal blood flow and glomerular filtration rate in the kidney leads to a decreased excretion of drugs that are eliminated renally.

Pharmacodynamic changes, which influence the onset, duration, and intensity of drug action or the response to a given dosage, are attributed to alterations occurring at organ system receptor sites. The central nervous system and cardiovascular system receptor sites are affected the most profoundly with regard to postural stability. Drug action is enhanced for most medications within the central nervous system, particularly for psychoactive drugs, because of degenerative changes in brain matter and the neurotransmitters. An increase in body sway or unsteadiness has been demonstrated to occur shortly after the administration of psychotropic medications. In the cardiovascular system, a decline in baroreflex activity increases the body's sensitivity to antihypertensive agents and contributes to the risk of postural hypotension.

Taken together, pharmacokinetic and pharmacodynamic alterations make older people susceptible to drug interactions and side effects that enhance the risk of falls and injury. The classes of medications associated most commonly with falls include diuretics, hypnotics and sedatives, antidepressants, psychotropics, and antihypertensives. Any of these drugs can interfere with postural control, motor and sensory coordination, or cognitive function, which may adversely influence gait and balance and induce a fall. Other medications, such as nonsteroidal anti-inflammatory agents (NSAIDs) and laxatives, have been implicated as a cause of falls. Their action is not direct but contributory, adding to the effects of underlying arthri-

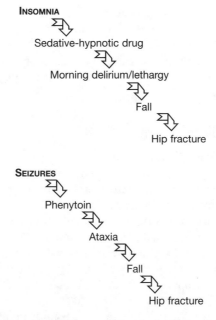

Figure 2-12. Example of medications prescribed for the treatment of medical problems such as insomnia and seizures and the potential side effects leading to falls and injury.

tis or a mobility dysfunction. Thus, older people may exceed their capabilities—for example, when rushing to the bathroom—and fall.

The risk of falling is greatest when taking drugs with extended half-lives (greater than 24 hours) and increases with the number of medications a person consumes. In principle, the risk of falls and injury should always be taken into consideration when medications are prescribed. Particular care must be taken with drugs that have the potential for adverse effects on cognitive function and/or gait and balance. Although these medications may be acceptable for treating the underlying problem, their side effects can increase the risk of falls and injury (Figure 2-12).

EXTRINSIC FACTORS

A number of extrinsic factors play an important role in fall causation. These factors consist of the physical environment, the design of furnishings, the condition of ground surfaces, and illumination. In addition, several devices used to promote mobility (e.g., walkers, wheelchairs) or guard against falls (e.g., mechanical restraints, bed side rails) have been implicated in causing falls. Also, the type and condition of footwear worn by patients and residents can play a primary role in fall causation.

Physical Environment

Most institutional falls experienced by older patients and residents occur in the bedroom, bathroom, and dining areas, reflecting the amount of time people spend in these areas.[6] In conjunction with patient- or resident-initiated activities, several environmental obstacles and design features are associated with falls: transferring from inappropriately low or high bed heights or climbing over bed side rails; sitting on and rising from low-seated, unstable, armless chairs and low-seated toilets lacking grab bar support; walking in poorly illuminated areas and tripping over low-lying objects or floor coverings, such as thick-pile carpeting and upended linoleum or tile flooring; and slipping on highly polished or wet ground surfaces and sliding rugs. The probability of the physical environment contributing to falls is highest for individuals with mobility problems (e.g., altered gait and balance, impaired transfers), wherein the physical demands of activities or tasks may exceed the competence of the individual.

Relocation—moving from home to hospital or nursing facility, from one facility to another, from hospital to nursing facility and vice versa, or from one hospital unit to another—can increase the risk of falls. New environments can affect frail older people adversely, particularly individuals with mobility problems. Also, people with dementia may not tolerate change well, increasing their confusion and their risk of falls. Relocation to a new environment, which includes unfamiliar surroundings; new roommates, social situations, and nursing and other staff; and changes in daily activities, can be stressful and potentially disorienting for people with dementia.

Devices

Devices such as mechanical restraints and, more often, side rails, are used with people who are at risk for falls in an attempt to protect them. It is ironic that these devices may actually increase fall risk in some instances. When patients or residents exit the bed by climbing over elevated bed side rails, perhaps catching their arms or legs in the rails, transferring activity becomes dangerous and increases fall risk (Figure 2-13). Also, individuals are more susceptible to injury, such as a fracture, when a

Figure 2-13. Transfers over elevated bed side rails can increase fall risk.

fall from a great height occurs. In addition, bed side rails are associated with a host of other injuries, such as soft-tissue bruises, contusions, lacerations, and fractures. These injuries result when people become entrapped in bed side rails, bump into rails, or fall between the mattress and bed side rail while attempting to get out of bed. Bed side rails have been known to break or become unhitched from bed frames during transfers. Most bed side rail injuries are associated with full-length rails. However, this statement does not imply that half side rails are benign (i.e., in some instances, half side rails are not sturdy enough to support safe bed transfers).

The use of mechanical restraints can contribute to falls. Older adults can untie or slip out of restraints when they are applied improperly. As a result, older adults can fall from chairs and wheelchairs or out of bed. Patients and residents also may become entangled in restraints while attempting to get out of bed. Using restraints may increase older adults' risk of falls because of the effects of immobilization caused by restraint devices (e.g., deconditioning, muscle weakness, loss of joint flexibility, vasomotor instability). In addition, restraints can lead to increased anxiety, anger, agitation, and confusion, which heighten risk for falls. Moreover, the effectiveness of mechanical restraints in preventing falls and related injuries is doubtful. Restrained patients and residents experience more falls and serious fall-related injuries than do unrestrained individuals. Institutions that have limited their use of mechanical restraints have experienced either no increase in falls or only a slight increase. Any increase in falls that may have resulted from eliminating restraints, however, has not been accompanied by an increase in serious fall-related injuries.

Canes and walkers, devices prescribed to support mobility, can contribute to unsafe mobility if they are the wrong size, are used improperly, or are in a poor state of repair (e.g., worn rubber tips, structural breakdown). Patients and residents with inappropriate or malfunctioning walking devices may abandon or use their ambulation aid sparingly, which increases the risk of falls. Wheelchairs contribute to falls when a poor transfer technique (i.e., not locking wheel brakes, feet not clearing the footplates) is used. Wheelchairs may roll away or tip over during transfers. At other times, poor wheelchair design (e.g., inaccessibility of wheelchair brakes; short handles, improper footrest placement) and the condition of the chair itself (e.g., broken equipment, worn brakes and footrests) can be responsible for falls. In addition, falls from wheelchairs sometimes occur when patients and residents reach for objects or lean too far forward in their chairs, leading to wheelchair instability. People with cognitive impairments and lower extremity problems are at special risk for wheelchair falls; for example, they do not remember to lock wheelchair brakes or they fail to clear the footplates when exiting the chair. Some individuals in wheelchairs who exhibit agitated behaviors may excessively rock their chairs to the point of tipping them over.

Footwear

Improper footwear can alter gait and balance and lead to falls. High-heeled shoes narrow the standing and walking base of support, decrease stride length, and place individuals in a forward-leaning posture, causing their balance to become precarious and making them susceptible to falls. Poorly fitting shoes, loose shoes in particular, can affect ambulation adversely. In an effort to keep their shoes on, people may shuffle when they walk, then trip. Leather-soled shoes promote slipping as does wearing socks without shoes. Rubber crepe soles, although slip-resistant, may stick to linoleum floor surfaces. Such sticking can halt gait precipitously, causing forward balance loss and falls, particularly in older adults with decreased foot–ground clearance. Thick-soled footwear such as running shoes or sneakers may decrease the proprioceptive feedback that is derived from striking the foot on the ground during ambulation and cause a loss of balance.

Situational Circumstances

Situational circumstances also are responsible for predisposing older adults to falls and for contributing to falls. The circumstances examined here are length of stay in the health care facility, time at which the fall occurs, and specific characteristics of the facility staff.

Length of Stay   Commonly, older adults fall during the first week and after the third week of institutional stay. Various explanations have been offered. Incidents during the first week may be attributable to lack of familiarity with the environment or the presence of acute (i.e., altered homeostasis) or chronic diseases (i.e., altered mobility). Hospital patients who are perceived by both themselves and the staff as ready for discharge after the third week may be more likely to fall because they have been allowed full mobility. Residents of nursing facilities with functional limitations requiring staff assistance at the time of admission can improve their functional status with restorative care and thus may be allowed independent freedom of movement. However, they may not have recovered their mobility fully, placing them at certain fall risk, which may account for falls after the third week. In acute care hospitals, increased length of stay is positively correlated with an increase in falls, presumably due to a greater chance of iatrogenic (i.e., induced inadvertently by a physician or by medical and/or surgical treatment, such as anesthetic effects) factors contributing to the risk.

Time of Fall   Most falls occur during the night (i.e., 11 P.M.–7 A.M.) and select daylight hours (i.e., 6 A.M.–10 A.M.; 4 P.M.–8 P.M.). The primary explanation for nocturnal falls has been that older people get up to toilet, despite the fact that their ability to transfer safely out of bed is diminished and that they travel to the bathroom under poor illumination conditions. Also contributing to fall risk is that there is less staff available at night and on weekends to assist patients and residents. The hours of peak frequency of falls during daylight hours correspond with heightened waking activity levels.

Staff Characteristics   Staffing patterns, the number of nurses and nursing assistants available on any one shift, may also influence fall occurrence. Most research shows an inverse correlation between falls and the number of staff available; falls increase as staff is decreased and as the number of staff increases, the frequency of falls declines. Sometimes the correlation is reversed; that is, falls increase with the addition of staff members. The reason for this reversed correlation is not entirely clear and may not relate strictly to the absolute number of nurses or to the ratio of staff to patients or residents, but rather to their availability and their attitudes toward assisting people who are mobility impaired. In other words, positive staff attitudes with respect to caring for older people may decrease the occurrence of falls, and negative attitudes may lead to acts of omission (e.g., failure to assess for risk and implement preventive strategies) and, thus, increased falls. Some have speculated that the presence of agency nurses may increase risk of falls on weekends (i.e., agency nurses may not be familiar with patients and residents under their care and may lack appropriate attitudes toward patient and resident safety). Therefore, falls may not be related to the number of staff or ratio of staff to patients or residents but instead to the availability of staff at the time of the fall and the attitudes of the staff. Other complicating factors include the location of the rooms of people who fall, particularly if patients or residents reside a long distance from the nurses' station and time-consuming trips by staff are required, and the number of staff present on different nursing shifts, weekends, and during holidays.

RISK FACTORS FOR FALLS AND INJURY

Although a number of intrinsic and extrinsic factors predispose older people to falls and injuries, the design of effective preventive measures is dependent on identifying the specific risk factors involved. Several host-related or intrinsic factors have been found repeatedly to be strongly associated with the risk of institutional falls:

- Decreased vision (e.g., cataracts, macular degeneration, glaucoma, hemianopsia)
- Lower extremity dysfunction (e.g., arthritis, muscle weakness, peripheral neuropathy, foot disorders)
- Gait/balance disorders (e.g., Parkinson's disease, stroke, cane/ walker use)
- Cardiovascular disorders (e.g., orthostatic hypotension, arrhythmia, syncope)

- Bladder dysfunction (e.g., nocturia, incontinence, frequency of urination)
- Cognitive/emotional dysfunction (e.g., dementia, depression, anxiety, fear of falling, denial of physical and functional limitations, refusal to use required assistive devices)
- Communication disorders (e.g., dysarthria, dysphasia)
- Medications (e.g., diuretics, antihypertensives, sedatives, psychotropics, NSAIDs, number of drugs or polypharmacy)

These factors, either in isolation or combination, contribute to altered mobility, the ability to achieve and maintain safe ambulation, transferring activities (e.g., on/off beds, chairs, toilets, wheelchairs), and bending/reaching activities (e.g., obtaining/placing objects; onto/ from nightstands; into/from closets, cabinets, dressers), or the ability to ask for required assistance with mobility tasks.

Diseases associated with lower extremity dysfunction contribute greatly to gait and balance problems. These diseases impair effective ambulation and the speed and reliability of postural reflexes to correct balance displacements. In addition, loss of lower extremity strength is significantly associated with transfer difficulties that arise when sitting on or rising from chairs, beds, and toilets. Visual disorders can impair the detection of ground surfaces or low-lying environmental objects and can interfere with the physiological compensation that corrects balance instability. Cognitive disturbances influence how an individual perceives and adapts to the environment and to activity demands. As a risk factor, urinary dysfunction is complex. Toileting requires people to rise from a bed or chair, ambulate to the bathroom, adjust their clothing, position themselves on the toilet, maintain their balance on the toilet, stand up, leave the bathroom, and return to the point of origin. A fall may occur at any time. In addition, there is a risk that on the way to the bathroom a person will become incontinent and slip in his or her urine. The synergistic effects of medications at inappropriate dosages and the overzealous use of hypnotic-anxiolytic agents contribute to gait and postural instability. The risk of falling increases with the number of intrinsic risk factors present; multiple risk factors are more likely to be present in individuals with recurrent falls than in people without recurrent falls. Furthermore, the risk of falls is greatly increased in patients and residents with a history of falls during the past 3 months and/or recurrent falls (i.e., multiple episodes occurring over a short period of time—days to weeks).

When these intrinsic risk factors are combined with undesirable environmental conditions or extrinsic factors, the risk of falling is increased further. For example, unsuitable environments such as low-seated furnishings and toilets, reduced illumination and hazardous ground surfaces may be negotiated easily by people who are functionally healthy. However, in individuals with altered mobility, the condition of the environment can be a major obstacle, leading to fall risk. The risk of injury following a fall is heightened by the presence of the following factors:

- Advanced age: Older women with osteoporosis are at particular risk
- Lower extremity weakness and loss of joint flexibility, and/or gait disturbances: Greater risk of balance loss and inability to recover balance
- Ambulation with a cane or walker: Increased likelihood of gait or balance disorder and fall risk
- Poor vision: Inability to detect ground surface hazards, which can lead to trips and slips
- Dementia: Errors in judgment between safe and hazardous tasks or the environment; reduced ability to correct imbalance
- Immobility: Increased probability of lower extremity weakness and joint inflexibility, resulting in balance loss and poor balance recovery

The risk of falls and injury occurs in three phases. Phase 1 is the initiating event that displaces the person's base of support and balance when walking. For patients and residents, these initiating events may be the result of lower extremity dysfunction such as muscle weakness, unstable joints, and diminished postural reflexes; or environmental hazards such as a slippery floor surface. Phase 2 occurs when the person's systems for maintaining upright posture or balance stability fail to recognize and correct the balance displacement in time to avoid a fall. Older people who fail to recover balance during falls may be experiencing a loss of sensory and motor functions, which may be the result of neurological and musculoskeletal disorders. Phase 3 of the fall, commonly referred to as the impact phase, occurs when the person hits the floor or other surface. It is during this phase that the forces of the impact are transmitted to the body, possibly resulting in an injury. Efforts to prevent falls and injury must begin at

Phase 1; the cause of falls must be evaluated and fall risk must be assessed, and subsequently, an attempt must be made to modify the risk factors discovered in an effort to prevent the occurrence of Phases 2 and 3. This approach is examined in the chapters that follow.

ENDNOTES

1. Janken, J.K., & Reynolds, B.A. (1987). Identifying patients with the potential for falling. In A. McLane (Ed.), *Classification of nursing diagnosis* (pp. 136–143). St. Louis: Mosby.
2. Myers, A.H., Baker, S.P., Van Natta, M.L., Abby, H., & Robinson, E.G. (1991). Risk factors associated with falls and injuries among elderly institutionalized persons. *American Journal of Epidemiology, 133,* 1179–1190.
3. Campbell, A.J. (1991). Drug treatment as a cause of falls in old age: A review of the offending agents. *Drugs and Aging, 1,* 289–302.
4. Ray, W.A., & Griffin, M.R. (1990). Prescribed medications and the risk of falling. *Topics in Geriatric Rehabilitation, 5,* 12–20.
5. Thapa, P.B., & Ray, W.A. (1996). Medications and falls and fall-related injuries in the elderly. In A.M. Bronstein, T. Brandt, & M.H. Woollacott (Eds.), *Clinical disorders of balance, posture and gait* (pp. 301–325). London: Arnold.
6. Connell, B.R. (1996). Role of the environment in falls prevention. *Clinics in Geriatric Medicine, 12(4),* 859–880.

clinical assessment and evaluation

The accumulated effects of multiple diseases, medications, and resulting disabilities, combined with extrinsic factors (i.e., environmental settings that are hazardous or unsuitable for safe mobility), predispose many older patients in hospitals and nursing facility residents to falls and subsequently cause them. However, the degree of individual fall risk and the etiology, or causes, of falls among older people varies considerably. Because of interindividual variability (e.g., differences in coexisting medical problems and their number and severity; the number, types, and dosages of medications used; the level of cognitive function and mobility capacity; design and structure of institutional environments), some people are at greater fall risk than others, and thus, the etiology of falls is different. Consequently, both the prediction of individual fall risk and the determination of fall etiology is difficult without a comprehensive systematic approach.

The primary aim of the clinical assessment is to identify people who are at risk for falls and, in those with falls, to discover the causative factors. Once these factors have been identified, a clinical evaluation is performed in order to design preventive or interventional strategies to reduce fall risk. The steps involved in the fall and fall risk assessment are outlined in Figure 3-1.

FALL ASSESSMENT

A falling episode should be followed by an evaluation and treatment of physical injury, life-threatening medical conditions, or both, that may have precipitated or followed the falling event. Any time a fall occurs, the patient or resident should not be moved or assisted in

Step 1
Patient or resident has fallen: Proceed to Step 2. If patient or resident has not fallen: Proceed to Step 4.

Step 2
Evaluate for physical injury and/or acute medical problems. Provide treatment as indicated.

Step 3
Obtain fall history, circumstances of incident.

Step 4
Review fall risk factors (medical, psychological, and functional histories).

Step 5
Obtain Peformance-Oriented Environmental Mobility Screen (POEMS).

Step 6
Perform physical examination.

Step 7
Obtain laboratory and diagnostic studies as indicated.

Step 8
List differential diagnosis of fall(s) and/or identified fall risk factors.

Step 9
Implement interventions to reduce fall risk.

Step 10
Monitor/follow-up to determine success of interventions.

Step 11
Repeat assessment if patient or resident continues to fall or experiences new falls. If no falls, proceed to Step 12.

Step 12
Repeat fall risk assessment on a regular basis.

Figure 3-1. Steps involved in the fall and fall risk assessments.

getting up from the floor until the possibility of injury has been eliminated. Also, any symptoms or signs of acute medical problems must be referred for medical attention immediately. An injury and medical emergency checklist that nurses can use as a referral tool is provided in Section Two, Part B.

Once the patient or resident is medically stable, a history of the circumstances surrounding the fall should be taken to help determine the differential diagnosis. Taking a history is analogous to inquiring

terminology

Differential diagnosis	Distinguishing between two or more diseases with similar symptoms by systematically comparing their signs and symptoms
Hypoglycemia	Low blood sugar
Orthostatic hypotension	Lowered blood pressure that occurs on rising to an erect position
Proprioception	Muscle and joint sensations of body's position in space
Syncope	Fainting; temporary unconsciousness

about any other medical symptoms such as abdominal pain or chest pain. To discover the etiology, a history of the circumstances should be obtained, as should descriptive information on the duration, severity, and location of the discomfort. Taking a fall history consists of asking the person about any symptoms experienced at the time of the fall or those occurring prior to the fall (e.g., dizziness, heart palpitations, loss of consciousness or balance, legs giving away, trips or slips) and for a description of the activity the person was engaged in at the time of the fall. Because older adults may have poor recollection of these events because of cognitive impairment, reports from nurses, other staff members, and family members who may have witnessed the fall can be helpful. In addition, the location, time (hour of the day) of the fall, and any injuries sustained should be documented.

Asking patients and residents to recount the circumstances of their falls provides valuable clues to the etiologies. For example, falls associated with rising from a bed or chair and experiencing symptoms of dizziness may point to orthostatic hypotension (for a definition of this and other terms related to the chapter, see the terminology sidebar above). An absence of symptoms may implicate the design, the height, or the stability of the bed or chair as a causative factor. If a person complains of tripping or slipping, the environment (e.g., hazardous ground surface camouflaged by poor lighting, wet floors, upended carpet edges or linoleum tiles) may be the precipitating cause, either by itself or in combination with an underlying gait disorder.

In addition, the history should include inquiry about previous falls and their circumstances. This inquiry helps to determine whether there is a pattern to the falls. The majority of people who fall repeatedly do so under similar circumstances. This kind of information, if not available from the patient or resident, may be gathered from a review of available past incident reports or medical records. It is equally important to solicit information about near-falls. Near-falls are events in which a person loses balance but manages to avert a fall to the ground by grabbing onto an environmental object such as the back of a chair, a headboard, or a table edge for support. (If the environmental object had not been available for support, the person probably would have suffered a fall to the ground.) Observational studies of older people residing in institutions have demonstrated that in the course of their daily activities, many frail individuals encounter an increased frequency of near-falls, which increases the risk of falling.[1]

Other questions that should be asked about previous falls include whether the person has experienced any physical injury or loss of self-confidence in performing activities, or, subsequently, has restricted his or her mobility in any way. A positive response to the latter may indicate a fear of subsequent falls.

A thorough history aimed at identifying the circumstances associated with falling represents the foundation of determining fall etiology because all subsequent evaluations are based, in part, on the information obtained. As such, the fall history (see Figure 3-2 for fall history components, represented by the acronym SPLATT) can be incorporated into existing hospital and nursing facility incident reports and thus becomes a standard part of any investigation of falls.

Symptoms experienced at time of fall(s)

Previous number of falls or near-falls

Location of fall(s)

Activity engaged in at time of fall(s)

Time (hour of day) of fall(s)

Trauma (physical, psychological) associated with fall(s)

Figure 3-2.   Fall history to be gathered on an individual, using the acronym SPLATT.

FALL RISK ASSESSMENT

The assessment of fall risk in older adult patients of hospitals and residents of nursing facilities begins with the identification of individual risk factors from the thorough history.

Identification of Individual Risk Factors

A thorough history can detect most people who are at high risk for falling. The individual taking the history should inquire about the occurrence of falls during the previous 3 months and the circumstances surrounding the fall(s) and review the medical history for conditions and medications that place patients or residents at risk. Individual fall risk factors include

- Visual impairment
- Postural hypotension
- Reduced lower extremity strength
- Impaired gait and balance
- Impaired mobility
- Use of ambulation assistive devices
- Bladder dysfunction
- Altered cognition
- Polypharmacy (taking four or more medications)
- Sedatives, psychotropics, hypnotics, and antihypertensive drugs

These factors, particularly when they occur simultaneously, have been associated repeatedly with fall risk; attempts to ascertain their presence should be included in the risk assessment of patients and residents. Although these factors by themselves increase susceptibility to falls, their relationship as a true measure of fall risk is more accurately reflected by their effects on an individual's ability to ambulate and transfer safely and independently in the living environment. Any impairment in gait and balance that results from these factors is a strong predictor of fall risk. Therefore, a performance-oriented environmental mobility screen (POEMS), which evaluates how competently patients and residents execute a number of positional changes and movements during their daily activities, should be obtained. (A blank, photocopiable master form is included in Part B of Section Two.)

Performance-Oriented Environmental Mobility Screen

POEMS constitutes the second step of the assessment of fall risk and is beneficial in identifying host-related situations and environmental conditions that cause dysmobility in people at fall risk. POEMS assesses the following performance items: balance maintained in sitting and rising from a chair, bed, and toilet; standing balance; ability to bend down from a standing position; and ability to ambulate in both the bedroom and bathroom. Transfer and ambulation maneuvers are tested with or without assistive devices as applicable. Testing the person's capacity to ambulate in different locations takes into account that the space limitations, ground surfaces, and illumination of the space are dissimilar and represent different risks. Individuals are scored on each task as being either normal (i.e., independent mobility) or impaired (i.e., person is unsteady during performance or unable to accomplish the task or perform the task safely). Any impaired execution indicates that the person is at fall risk.

Depending on the patient's or resident's state of health during time of admission and institutional stay, the sequence of POEMS maneuvers may be altered to accommodate the individual. In patients and residents who are ill, the length of the POEMS is determined by the individual's capacity to continue performing the maneuver safely. The list below suggests sequences for people who are ill and for people who are well.

Illness

- Transfer off bed
- Stand after rising from bed (eyes open)
- Stand with eyes closed
- Stand in place (sternal nudge)
- Bend down, pick up object
- Walk around bedroom/bed
- Walk to/around bathroom
- Sit down/rise from toilet
- Walk up/down hallway
- Transfer onto bed

Wellness

- Sit down/rise from chair

- Stand after rising from chair (eyes open)
- Stand with eyes closed
- Stand in place (sternal nudge)
- Bend down, pick up object
- Transfer onto/off bed
- Walk around bedroom/bathroom
- Sit down on/rise from toilet
- Walk up/down hallway

POEMS is initiated in the older person's bedroom. The individual is asked to sit down and rise from a chair. The person doing the screening should observe the person's ability to complete the activity in a smooth and controlled movement, without loss of balance or the use of armrests. The chair should not tip or slide away and the person's feet should not slide but rest flat on the floor (Figure 3-3). Next, the person should be instructed to rise from the chair and remain standing in place for approximately 30 seconds. The person doing the screening should observe whether the person is able to stand without loss of balance or support from the chair to maintain balance (Figure 3-4). The person should be asked to participate in the Romberg test, which assesses proprioceptive function: He or she should remain standing with eyes closed, arms placed at his or her sides, and feet planted approximately 3 inches apart. Inability to maintain balance, as demonstrated by increased postural sway or grabbing environmental furnishings for support, indicates an abnormality (Figure 3-5).

A sternal push test should be performed by the examiner with the person standing still with his or her eyes open. The push test

Figure 3-3. Chair transfer.

Figure 3-4. Immediate standing balance.

Figure 3-5. Romberg test.

consists of nudging the person's sternum lightly with the fingers while applying enough force to induce balance displacement (Figure 3-6). This maneuver tests postural competence in response to loss of balance. The normal reaction is to stretch the arms forward, away from the body, and to take one or two steps backward (Figure 3-7). Both movements represent the body's ability to compensate for sudden balance shifts. The inability to maintain balance (e.g., a fall backward) signifies an abnormality (Figure 3-8).

During these postural tests, it is prudent for another staff member to be positioned behind the person in the event of a fall. In extremely frail individuals or in those who, from appearances, would obviously have difficulty recovering from imbalances, the sternal push test may be omitted for safety reasons.

Following the body displacement tests, the person should be asked to bend from a normal standing position as if to retrieve an object from the floor. The examiner should observe whether the person is steady and able to maintain balance without holding onto furnishings for support (Figure 3-9). The person's reaching activities, such as obtaining clothing from closets and other storage areas used by the individual, can be examined in a similar fashion.

Next, the person should be asked to transfer onto and off of the bed. The person's ability to perform this maneuver smoothly and

Figure 3-6. Sternal push test.

Figure 3-7. A normal reaction to body displacement.

Figure 3-8. An abnormal reaction to body displacement.

Figure 3-9. Bending-down performance.

controlled without loss of balance or need for arm support to maintain sitting balance on the mattress should be observed and rated. Also, the bed should remain steady (i.e., without moving or sliding away). The older person's feet should rest flat on the floor in the seated position (Figure 3-10).

The next performance item tests ambulation ability. The person should be asked to walk about and turn around, first in the bedroom and then in the bathroom, using the ambulation device if applicable. The examiner should observe the person's gait and balance, whether the person's gait is continuous and whether it occurs without hesitation or excessive deviation from side to side; whether both of the person's feet clear the surface of the floor; whether any incidences of staggering or losing balance and grabbing environmental surfaces (e.g., bed, chair backs, sink edge, walls) for support take place; and whether the ambulation device is used safely and fits into spaces (e.g., both sides of the bed, in the bathroom) (Figure 3-11).

Toilet transfer is the next area to be tested in POEMS. The person should be asked to transfer onto and off of the toilet. As with other tests, the person should be observed for his or her ability to perform this activity in a smooth, controlled movement, without loss of balance or the need to hold onto the sink edge or grab bars for support (Figure 3-12). Finally, the person should walk from the bedroom and

Figure 3-10. Bed transfer.

Figure 3-11. Common environmental walking routes are reflected by the shaded areas. A person should be able to use his or her ambulation device safely in all areas.

Figure 3-12. Toilet transfer.

down the hallway to the nurses' station and other locations, such as the dining room. The person should be observed for his or her ability to walk without gait and balance difficulties or fatigue.

If the person's POEMS results are normal (i.e., the patient or resident is able to perform the maneuvers independently), the person is at low fall risk. However, any impairment in execution of a task indicates the presence of underlying intrinsic and/or extrinsic factors (Table 3-1) that place the individual at fall risk.

Advantages of POEMS   POEMS has several advantages: It is easy to understand and administer by nurses and nursing assistants in both hospital and nursing facility settings. In general, it takes no longer than 10 minutes to complete, even with the frailest people. In addition to detecting mobility dysfunction, POEMS also can be used to help design rehabilitative and environmental interventions and to monitor clinical changes or outcomes (e.g., the effects of medical conditions, medications, environmental influences) over time.

Administering POEMS   Optimally, the fall risk assessment should be completed when people are first admitted to the hospital or nursing facility because the risk of falling is greatest during the first few days of institutional stay. However, completing the assessment may not always be feasible or practical, particularly in an acute care hospital. On admission to an acute care facility, patients may be injured (e.g., hip fracture) or severely ill. Often, people with rapidly fluctuating medical conditions are maintained by bed rest. In these instances, risk assessment is best administered after any acute problem or condition is treated and stabilized or at a time when the patient is permitted to assume an independent level of function. In both hospitals and nursing facilities, risk should be reassessed whenever the person's medical condition, medication regimen (e.g., the addition or subtraction of drugs, dosage modifications) and functional status change.

In nursing facilities and certain hospital units such as psychiatric wards, where people reside for prolonged periods of time, risk as-

Table 3-1. POEMS differential diagnoses

Impaired maneuver	Intrinsic factors	Extrinsic factors
Chair, bed, and toilet transfers	Parkinsonism Arthritis Deconditioning Adverse drug effects	Poor chair, bed, or toilet design
Standing balance	Postural hypotension Vestibular dysfunction Adverse drug effects	
Romberg test	Proprioceptive dysfunction Adverse drug effect	Poor illumination Overly absorptive footwear, carpeting, or both
Sternal push	Parkinsonism Normal pressure hydrocephalus Adverse drug effects	
Bending down	Central nervous system dysfunction Adverse drug effects	
Walking/turning	Foot disorders Parkinsonism Hemiparesis Sensory dysfunction Adverse drug effects	Improper footwear Improper size/use of ambulation device Hazardous ground surfaces

sessment, particularly POEMS, should be repeated at established intervals—approximately every 3–6 months. This should be done so as to identify people with gradually deteriorating health conditions because any decline in mobility can indicate an early sign of disease and fall risk.

POEMS can be incorporated into the Minimum Data Set 2.0 (MDS 2.0; Long-Term Care Facility Resident Assessment Instrument) in nursing facilities as follows:

MDS Full Assessment Form
    Section G: Physical Functioning and Structural Problems
    Bed mobility

Transfer
Walk in room
Walk in corridor
Locomotion on unit
Toilet use
Test for balance
Modes of locomotion
Modes of transfer
Change in activities of daily living (ADLs) function

MDS Quarterly Assessment Form
Section G1: ADL Performance
Bed mobility
Walk in room
Walk in corridor
Toilet use
Modes of transfer

Resident Assessment Protocols
Failure to thrive
ADLs
Functional Rehabilitation Potential
Falls
Psychotropic drug-related side effects (unsteady gait/balance)

Physical Restraints (risk of falls)

A fall risk checklist is presented in Part B of Section Two that can be used to help identify and record individual risk factors. In addition, the checklist can be incorporated into existing institutional examination forms, medical and nursing records, and incident reports. Once a patient or resident is identified as being at fall risk, all staff must be alerted. A number of measures have been used by nursing staff to recognize individuals at risk: application of brightly colored stickers placed on the medical and nursing charts, bedroom door, and bedside; and distinctively colored wrist identification bands or slippers to be worn by the person at risk.

Several hospitals and nursing facilities have developed standard fall risk assessment tools that predict a person's susceptibility to falls (see Bibliography). The sources of data used to develop these risk profiles vary greatly (e.g., incident report data, literature reviews of risk factors, staff experiences). A number of potential problems with these risk assessment tools have been identified. Staff members have varied definitions of a fall they report; some institutions may require only those falls resulting in physical injury to be reported; profiles developed from the literature are often skewed toward characteristics of a particular institution, hospital, or nursing facility; and within each institution, specific factors derived from specialized units (e.g., oncology, orthopedic, surgery, psychiatric, rehabilitation, neurology, stroke, dementia-specific care) may not apply to different institutions or settings.

Staffing patterns and environmental designs also may affect fall risk; indeed, in some instances they may constitute a greater determinant of risk than the characteristics of patients or residents by themselves. The most effective procedure is to examine the risk assessment tools available and choose several that seem to reflect the particular population of the facility. Each procedure should be used in a pilot program within hospital units and nursing facility floors that have a high incidence of falls. Their success is measured by assessing a group of people who have experienced falls and comparing them with a group of people without falls. Using the tool in this way should determine whether it is sensitive enough to differentiate fall risk. Questions that should be answered while using the tool include the following: Does the tool work? Does it accurately identify patients and residents at risk for falling? Is the tool practical? Do nurses find the instrument user-friendly for routine use? Being able to accurately identify patients and residents at risk on a regular basis enables resources (e.g., nursing and rehabilitative staff, safety equipment, assistive devices) to be targeted toward prevention.

CLINICAL EVALUATION

Once the falls and fall risk assessments have been completed, multiple fall etiologies and risk factors may be identified via clinical evaluation. The primary aim of the clinical evaluation is twofold: First, in people with a fall or falls, it isolates a specific cause; in people with identifiable risk factors, it uncovers the presence of remedial or modifiable factors. Second, the clinical evaluation determines in both groups the existence of any new risk factors that may not have been detected previously. Although, in general, the clinical evaluation is the province of physicians, allied health professionals (e.g., physicians' assistants, nurse practitioners, clinicians) are equally adept in assessment techniques. The services of these professionals are useful, particularly in the nursing facility, where the presence of physicians is rare.

The clinical evaluation of patients and residents with falls begins with a review of the medical records, current medical problems, and medications. This review may provide important clues to the factors contributing to falls. For example, if a person experiences dizziness prior to a fall and records indicate the recent addition of a diuretic to the person's medicines, the association of the two factors may indicate that the fall has been caused by an adverse medication effect. Similarly, if a person has arthritis in the knees and falls while transferring from a chair, the arthritis may be partially responsible for the fall.

Once the person's historical information is compiled, a POEMS should be obtained. As in people at fall risk, the value of POEMS for people who have fallen lies in isolating organ systems and environmental problems that may provide insight into the possible etiology of the fall. The next step is to perform a physical examination that includes comprehensive cognitive, neurological, musculoskeletal, and cardiac evaluations. Information gathered from the falls/fall-risk assessments and POEMS can serve as a focus for the physical examination. For example, if the fall history reveals that a fall occurred in association with dizziness and changes in position and POEMS demonstrates a loss of balance, unsteadiness, and/or the complaint of dizziness on immediate standing, postural changes in blood pressure must be assessed to rule out or confirm orthostatic hypotension. Similarly, if the person demonstrates difficulty with chair or bed transferring during POEMS, the physical examination should concentrate on evaluating the musculoskeletal system for reduced muscle strength. Not only will any abnormality discovered during the physical examination help to identify the cause of falls and modifiable risk factors but also other, not-directly-related findings, which may increase the risk of subsequent falls, may be detected.

Once the physical examination has been completed, the next step is to perform laboratory and diagnostic studies. The extent of

Figure 3-13. The fall-risk assessment pathway. This assessment should be repeated regularly to identify new or changing risk factors.

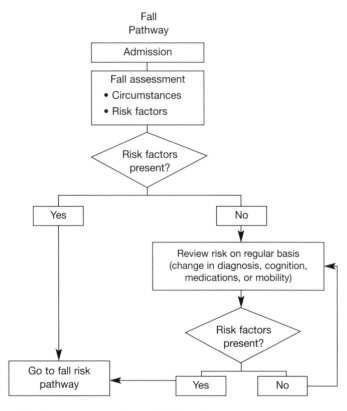

Figure 3-14. The fall assessment and evaluation pathway.

testing is dictated by the information gathered from all previous evaluations. For example, if the physical examination confirms the presence of orthostatic hypotension, blood and stool testing for volume-depleted states such as dehydration, blood loss, and anemia must be ordered. If the person is diabetic and the history suggests falls resulting from hypoglycemia, a blood glucose test should be obtained. If the fall is associated with a syncopal episode and the physical examination reveals an irregular pulse rate, an electrocardiogram and possibly a Holter monitoring study should be considered. A history of bladder dysfunction demands urine and blood tests and urodynamic studies to search for underlying causes. Similarly, manifestations of lower extremity weakness on physical examination indicate the need for tests that may explain the etiology.

After all evaluations are complete, a list of intrinsic or extrinsic (or both) factors responsible for fall risk or falls can be compiled. From the list(s), interventions to reduce the risk of subsequent falls should follow (see Chapter 4). Follow-up ensures that the intervention strategies employed are effective. Repeat the fall-risk assessment by using flowcharts or pathways, as shown in Figures 3-13 and 3-14, on a regular basis to identify new or changing risk factors (Figure 3-13). If the person continues to fall, repeat the fall assessment and evaluation (Figure 3-14). Some factor may have been missed or overlooked from previous evaluations, or the person may have developed an additional condition that causes falls. It is important to remember that falls and fall risk are not fixed or static processes but rather are dynamic events, and the causes can change as often as do the person's medical conditions and environmental surroundings.

ENDNOTE

1. Connell, B.R., & Wolf, S.L. (1993). Patterns of naturally occurring falls among frail nursing home residents. *Gerontologist*, *33*(Special Issue), 58.

preventive strategies to reduce fall risk

The goal of fall prevention strategies is to design interventions that minimize fall risk by ameliorating or eliminating contributing factors while maintaining or improving patients' and residents' mobility. Potential preventive strategies are based on known risk factors and postulated causes of falls and can be classified as medical, rehabilitative, and environmental. In most cases, management of people at fall risk includes components derived from each category. Although little direct evidence exists on the effectiveness of any one of these particular approaches in preventing falls, common sense suggests that they are promising and should be attempted. A description of these measures designed to prevent or reduce the incidence of falls, which can be used by hospital and nursing facility staff, along with an elaboration of fall prevention programs developed in institutional settings, follows.

MEDICAL STRATEGIES

The importance of identifying patients and residents at fall risk and those with falls and following up with a clinical evaluation of each to identify modifiable factors cannot be overemphasized. Each factor may represent a sign or symptom of an underlying disease or medication effect that requires a clinician's attention in order to rule out reversible acute problems, identify chronic medical conditions that may contribute, and treat each appropriately. Of equal importance is the assessment of medications. All drugs should be reviewed carefully in terms of their risks and benefits. Dosages should be examined with an eye toward reduction when possible. Any combination of drugs

should be monitored on a regular basis for potential drug interactions. In particular, drugs that affect mobility or increase fall risk
such as sedatives, hypnotics, and psychoactives should be scrutinized
routinely. As a general rule, medications in older people should be initiated
at their lowest effective dose, increased slowly while monitoring for
side effects and clinical efficacy, maintained at the lowest possible dose,
and discontinued when no longer effective. For patients and residents
with osteoporosis who are at risk for injurious falls, consideration of
drug treatment (e.g., calcium supplements and medications that reduce bone loss) to modify the risk of hip and other fractures is advised.

REHABILITATIVE STRATEGIES

Patients and residents who fail to respond or improve with medical
treatment and continue to remain at fall risk, particularly those with
chronic neuromuscular disorders, may respond to a number of rehabilitative strategies. These strategies include engaging in exercise
therapy, wearing proper footwear, employing hip-protective pads, and
using appropriate ambulation devices to assist with mobility.

Exercise

People with impaired muscular strength and altered gait and balance—
the consequences of underlying medical conditions, deconditioning,
or both—may benefit from low-intensity leg strengthening and
weight-bearing exercises as well as gait, balance, and transfer training generally provided by physiatrists and physical therapists. These
kinds of exercise and training programs are designed to restore and
maintain muscle strength and coordination, bone mass, joint flexibility and movement, vestibular and proprioceptive function, and
postural control reflexes, as well as to teach individuals effective bed,
chair, and toilet transfer techniques. In addition, there are a variety
of exercise programs that nurses and nursing assistants can easily
perform on their own to help maintain patient and resident mobility
(see Table 4-1). Figure 4-1 illustrates a set of simple exercises designed to maintain or improve mobility. These exercises can be per-

Table 4-1. Types of ambulation programs

Daily Floor Ambulation Program

Ambulatory patients or residents are encouraged to walk at least three times daily, or 30–45 minutes a day as tolerated, to the dining room, planned activities, and so forth. Assistance with ambulation is provided for individuals with poor gait and balance and/or fear of falling. The use of wheelchairs is discouraged.

"Walkers Group"

Ambulatory patients or residents are encouraged to walk daily from bed to bathroom, from bedroom to nurses' station, from bedroom to the end of the hallway, from one end of the hallway to the other end, and so forth, with set goals determined by physical condition. Rewards are given for achieving each goal.

Wheelchair Walking Program

Patients or residents are encouraged to "walk" with their chairs—to move their wheelchairs along by using their legs. This exercise helps them to maintain effective and safe transfers and improves lower extremity function. Removing the footrests discourages their use.

Mobility Program

Patients or residents are encouraged to ambulate and/or stand at least three times daily and to walk to the activity room for group exercises and meals daily. Patients, residents, and/or their caregivers are taught active and passive range-of-motion exercises, weight-bearing exercises, and resistive and aerobic exercises.

formed by staff either at the person's bedside or in a group setting, depending on the institution. These exercises should be started gradually and be done twice daily. The facilitator should work at the patient's or resident's own pace and level of stability. (Strength building can be intensified by adding 1- to 2-pound weights when performing Exercises 2 and 3.) For most patients and residents, these exercise therapy programs pose a minimal risk of adverse effects (i.e., injury), and they may be effective in combating impaired mobility and decreasing the risk of falls and injury.

A growing body of evidence suggests that older people respond to exercise therapy, even those who are very old and frail. Exercise can enhance the functioning of other organ systems involved in mobility endurance, such as cardiovascular and pulmonary performance. In addition, by building patients' and residents' self-confidence in performing activities, fear of falling or instability may be reduced. Because these individuals may be susceptible to falls and injury, caution

Exercise 1: Chair Rise/Sit (improves lower extremity strength and joint motion)

Ask the patient or resident to stand up from a stable chair and then sit down. If necessary, the patient or resident should use the armrest of the chair for support. 8–10 reps, as tolerated.

Exercise 2: Modified Sit-Up (improves lower extremity strength and joint motion)

Ask the patient or resident to lift each leg from the knee. 6–8 reps, as tolerated.

Exercise 3: Standing Knee Bend (improves lower extremity strength and balance)

Ask the patient or resident to lift leg, bend, and straighten at knee. Alternate right and left legs. 10 reps, as tolerated.

Figure 4-1.   Flexibility and balance exercise program.

Exercise 4: Shoulder Shrug (improves upper extremity range of motion)

Ask the patient or resident to sit up or stand up straight, shrug the shoulders up high, and release. 10 reps, as tolerated.

Exercise 5: Arm Circles (improves upper extremity range of motion)

Ask the patient or resident to sit up or stand up straight. With each arm make a circle, which gradually increases to become as large as possible. Begin the exercise with the arms 6 inches from sides and circle arms upward and down again. Each circle, 20 seconds; 2 reps, as tolerated.

Exercise 6: Ankle Pumps (improves ankle strength and balance)

Ask the patient or resident to lift up body on tiptoes and lower body back down while holding on to the back of a stable chair. This exercise may be done in a chair if the patient or resident has poor balance: Ask the individual to lift up heels on tiptoes and lower the heels back down again. 15 reps, as tolerated.

Figure 4-2. Assisted ambulation using a gait belt.

is advised—a renewed sense of confidence and ability to execute mobility tasks may lead these individuals to attempt activities that exceed their capabilities. This possibility should not dissuade staff from encouraging patient and resident independence in mobility, however. Instead, individuals should receive assistance at the beginning of such a program, and the assistance should continue until the individual can participate in the activities safely and independently.

For people who fall, mobility should be encouraged as soon as possible in order to avoid the consequences of immobility. If patients or residents require assistance with walking, nursing staff can make use of a gait belt (Figure 4-2). The belt serves as a ready "handle" to grasp in the event that the older person begins to fall. Staff should hold on to the belt handles or the tail strap with one hand and, with the other hand, hold on to the person's shoulder, which helps to control balance if the older person falls forward or backward. If the patient or resident does lose balance, the staff member should maintain normal posture (i.e., should not bend over): The knees should be bent, with the feet spaced 12 inches apart. The person should be pulled gently toward the staff member, or his or her descent to the ground controlled gently. Some staff and even the older person may find that a gait belt provides added security. To assist an individual walking without a cane, the staff member should position him- or herself in back and slightly to the side of the individual. If the individual uses a cane or hemiwalker, the staff member should stand on the opposite side of the device. To ensure safety, the patient or resident should never be pushed beyond safe limits—the activity should be stopped if the individual complains of fatigue or if gait and balance become unsafe. It is also a good idea to consult with a physical therapist on proper techniques for assisted walking.

Footwear

All footwear—shoes and slippers worn by patients and residents—
should fit properly and have slip-resistant soles. If foot problems
such as hammertoes, bunions, calluses, and nail disorders prohibit
the wearing of proper-sized shoes, individuals should be referred for
podiatric care. To accommodate foot problems, individuals may be
prescribed special therapeutic footwear (i.e., "Frankenstein" shoes).
Some frail older people may experience difficulty walking in this
type of shoe, which can increase fall risk. The shoes are somewhat
heavy to wear, and, as a result, the person may shuffle when walking,
which can lead to tripping. Cutting out the toe box of the shoes may
be a good alternative to therapeutic footwear, which interferes with
safe walking.

Shoes and slippers with rubber or crepe soles provide adequate
slip resistance on linoleum floors. Socks with nonskid tread on the
soles (Figure 4-3) are a good choice, par-
ticularly for people who make nocturnal
bathroom trips. However, for some individuals, such as those with a shuffling gait
or poor steppage height (i.e., inability to
pick up the feet an adequate distance from
the floor), slip-resistant soles may interfere with safe ambulation because the soles
adhere to ground surfaces. In particular,
disposable foam "hospital slippers" and
sneakers or running shoes with thick rubber soles can adhere to the
ground surface when an individual is walking in them. For such individuals, footwear with leather-type soles that promote gliding on linoleum and carpeted floor surfaces may be a better choice in institutional settings having a mixture of floor surfaces (i.e., both linoleum
and carpeting); however, a certain amount of caution in the selection
of soles is suggested. For some older people, footwear with smooth
soles (lack of traction) can facilitate walking on carpeted surfaces but
promotes slipping when walking on linoleum-covered surfaces.

Footwear with thick, soft soles may interfere with proprioceptive feedback (i.e., it may cause an inability to "feel" the ground while
walking), resulting in a loss of balance. Wearing thin, hard rubber-

Figure 4-3. Socks with nonskid tread soles.

soled shoes (e.g., boat shoes, Topsiders) can help a person preserve his or her balance. The best way to evaluate the adequacy of the sole surface of footwear is to observe patients and residents as they walk on different floor surfaces in their environment to see whether their footwear interferes with safe ambulation.

High-heeled shoes should be avoided because they narrow a person's standing and walking base of support, which can lead to a loss of balance. Footwear with low, broad heels is a better choice and should be encouraged. These shoes are better suited for safe walking and balance. However, if the patient or resident insists on wearing high heels—either out of vanity or because of a real need—she should be cautioned that high heels worn over a long period of time cause a shortening of the Achilles tendon, which then necessitates their use. Staff should then encourage the wearing of shoes with wedge heels (Figure 4-4). Wedge heels provide a better base of support than ordinary high-heeled shoes, and they are less likely to catch on an elevated floor surface, such as upended carpet, linoleum tile edges, or door thresholds.

Figure 4-4.   Shoes with wedge heels.

Hip-Padding Systems

More than 90% of hip fractures in older people are related to direct trauma against a hard ground surface following a fall. Hip-padding systems (Figure 4-5) are designed to act as shock absorbers around the hip (i.e., providing a cushion between the hip bone and impact surface), diverting the direct impact of a fall away from the bone, which helps to reduce the risk of a hip fracture. Three different types of hip-padding systems are available:

1.   Thin, elliptical plastic shields either sewn into specially designed undergarments or placed into pockets inside an ordinary pair of underwear; the shields are positioned to cover the hip bone
2.   Two shock-absorbent foam pads inserted into a lightweight wraparound garment that is worn under outer clothing and over

underwear; Velcro closures are used to allow for easy application and removal of the system

3. Adhesive pads made of flexible cork that fix directly to the skin over the hip area; the pads are designed to be left in place for several days

Figure 4-5. Example of a hip padding system (Hip-Guard). (Illustration reproduced with the permission of Prevent-Wise, Inc.)

Hip-padding systems can factor significantly in preventing hip fractures and have demonstrated benefits for both nursing facility residents and hospital patients.[1, 2] However, questions remain as to who should wear hip pads, how to convince individuals to wear them, and what kinds of hip pads are the most effective.

Approximately 50%–80% of older people comply with hip protectors, wearing them regularly. Compliance is higher in individuals who are cognitively intact and in people who have recently experienced an injurious fall. A fear of falling improves a person's initial acceptance of hip protectors, perhaps because they offer the individual a psychological peace-of-mind benefit. Therefore, hip-padding systems may be most helpful as a preventive strategy against hip fractures in select groups of patients and residents such as those at risk for further hip fracture and those with a fear of falling or injury.

Individuals' noncompliance with wearing hip pads seems to fall in one of two types: either initial rejection—the person does not want to wear hip pads—or later rejection—the person initially accepts wearing hip pads, but subsequently refuses to wear them. Several factors are associated with noncompliance, including altered cognitive status and wearability.

Altered Cognitive Status Patients and residents with dementia may lack the capacity to comprehend or recognize the need for hip protectors or they may become agitated while wearing the pads, forcing their removal. It is important to remember that not all people with dementia think about or respond to situations similarly; thus, some individuals reject hip pads or become disturbed by their presence, whereas other people accept and use hip protectors without complaint. In general, people with severe dementia are more tolerant of hip pads than are individuals with mild to moderate dementia. Because people with dementia are at significant risk for falling (e.g., from participating in hazardous activities, from not asking for assistance with activities, from developing small-stepped gaits) and fracturing their hips, attempts to provide hip protectors to people with mild to moderate dementia should not be abandoned. Some patients and residents, especially those with dementia, may need to have the purpose of the hip protector explained to them each time it is applied in order to circumvent agitation.

Wearability   Some older individuals complain that hip protectors are uncomfortable to wear, that they are too bulky when sitting in chairs or while sleeping in bed, that they are too hot or tight to wear under clothing, and that they are too difficult to remove in readiness for toileting (this is especially the case in those individuals with urinary incontinence and frequency). Staff members sometimes complain that hip protectors are difficult to care for, particularly in people who are incontinent, and/or are too difficult to remove when assisting incontinent individuals with scheduled toileting regimens. Alternatives that increase compliance include

- Selecting times when hip protectors are worn (e.g., days when individuals feel more unsteady) or not worn (e.g., during sleep, although nocturia, or excessive urination at night, is a risk factor for falls)
- Asking individuals to wear pants and dresses that are a few sizes larger than usual (to accommodate hip pads)
- Providing soft-seated chairs, which may be more comfortable for people to sit in

Studies assessing the effectiveness of the different hip-padding systems in reducing hip fractures and increasing wearability are in progress. It is, therefore, too early to recommend any hip-padding system over the others with certainty. However, because sometimes the point of impact following a fall is not directly on the hip but on the buttock, the foam-padding system, which wraps around the pelvis, may offer more protection than the plastic shield system. The wrap-around foam-padding system may protect against hip fracture in frail individuals with osteoporosis and poor balance who are constantly bumping against hard surfaces, such as walls and table edges. In addition, staff may find the foam-padding system easier to use in people who are incontinent because it can be used in conjunction with adult incontinence pads. Because hip-padding systems used by themselves cannot preclude the possibility of an individual's sustaining a hip fracture, hip protectors alone cannot be relied on in the prevention of fractures but must be used in conjunction with other preventive efforts.

Ambulation Devices

Ambulation devices, such as canes or walkers, are designed to improve gait and balance and to decrease the risk of falls. They work by creating greater stability, which increases an individual's standing and walking base of support because they provide an additional point or points of ground contact (Figure 4-6). Ambulation devices furnish proprioceptive feedback through the handles and reduce the load on weight-bearing joints, such as hips and knees. Also, devices provide individuals with visual physical support, which instills confidence in people during ambulation, helping to reduce their fear of instability and falls.

The choice of a cane, whether single- or multistemmed, or a walker, whether pick-up or wheeled type, should be determined by

| Two-legged stance, no ambulation device | Stance with standard cane (right-handed) | Stance with standard walker |

Figure 4-6. Base of support (shaded areas) provided by ambulation devices.

each individual's needs (see Table 4-2 for a list of types of assistive ambulation devices). In some ways, ambulation devices should be treated as medications: They should be "prescribed" to correct a specific underlying gait and balance problem and, as a consequence, tailored to fit both the person and the environment. Also, individuals must be instructed in the proper use of the device in walking and transferring in order to prevent adverse effects, such as falls and subsequent injury; this is best accomplished by referring patients and residents to a physiatrist or physical therapist.

Despite best efforts to prescribe the correct device and instruct individuals in using an assistive device properly, many patients and residents use ill-fitting devices and/or use them inappropriately, which heightens the risk of falls. Nurses and other hospital and facility staff are in a position to detect errors at an early stage and to decrease fall risk through corrective intervention. Corrective intervention can be accomplished by first ensuring that canes and walkers are the appropriate size (for an explanation of measurement techniques, see Ambulation Device Measurement Guidelines in Part A of Section Two), and, second, ensuring that patients and residents are using their devices properly during activities (see Ambulation Device Utilization Guidelines in Section Two for suggestions on how to help individuals use devices when walking, standing, turning, or sitting). In addition to checking for the proper size or fit and correct use of devices, ambulation devices should be inspected routinely for defects (see Table 4-3). Inspection is of particular importance in nursing facilities, where the mobility status and device requirements of residents are likely to change over time.

Wheelchairs

Wheelchairs are designed for patients and residents with limited ability to walk or who are totally dependent in walking. Wheelchairs come in a variety of sizes, designs, and materials, all of which are determined by the needs of the patient or resident. It is essential for nursing and other staff to work with physical and occupational therapists to ensure proper chair selection, fit, and use. The problems most commonly causing wheelchair falls and suggestions on how to correct them are described in the Wheelchair Problems and Modifications Checklist in Part B of Section Two.

Table 4-2. Types of assistive ambulation devices

Standard Cane

The standard cane is the most commonly used ambulation device. It is shaped like a candy cane and is usually made of wood or adjustable aluminum. The crook handle of the standard cane decreases grip strength, particularly in individuals with arthritis. The point of support is in the front of the hand, which makes this cane slightly unsteady. The cane should be held in the hand opposite to the disability (e.g., if pain is in right knee, cane is held in left hand). For balance support, however, the cane may be held in either hand.

Ortho Cane

The ortho cane is made of aluminum and is adjustable. It is similar to the standard cane. The shaft of the cane is offset, thereby placing the point of support directly below the handle. This design offers more stability than does the standard cane. The handle is molded, which provides a more comfortable grip than the standard cane.

Quad Cane

The quad cane has four legs and is used by individuals with impairment or weakness in one leg but who possess adequate balance control. This cane is more stable than the standard cane. It comes in a variety of base sizes. Base size is important because the wider the base, the greater the stability. Individuals with dementia may experience difficulty with quad canes. If the handle is not held facing the proper direction, the cane becomes very unstable, leading to loss of balance. Also, people with impaired vision may easily trip over the legs of the cane.

Hemi-Walker

The hemi-walker is a one-arm walker with four legs. This walker offers more support than the quad cane due to its broadly based legs. It is designed for individuals who are unable to use a standard walker (e.g., a hemiplegic with only one functioning upper extremity). Use of the hemi-walker requires good balance control and upper arm strength to move the walker.

Standard Walker

The standard walker consists of four adjustable legs equipped with rubber tips. The walker is designed for individuals with poor balance and lower extremity weakness or impairment. Walkers may be either nonfolding or folding. Nonfolding walkers offer greater stability and may be more appropriate than folding walkers for people living in long-term care facilities.

The device itself has several limitations: The individual using the walker must pick up the walker while walking, which results in a loss of balance when all four legs of the walker are off the floor. Individuals with poor balance and/or upper extremity weakness may push the device along the floor, causing the walker to suddenly halt and tip over, a particular problem on carpeted floor coverings. Applying metal furniture tips to the legs can overcome this problem, although the walker may slide away from some individuals.

(continued)

Table 4-2.   *(continued)*

Rolling Walker

The rolling walker is similar in design to the standard walker; however, it is equipped with either two front wheels or wheels attached to all four legs. The rolling walker does not require lifting and, therefore, is suited for individuals with poor balance and limited upper extremity strength. The two-wheeled walker is difficult to move on carpeted floor coverings because the rear legs drag along the floor; applying metal furniture tips to the rear legs overcomes this problem. The four-wheel walker is easier to move along, but may roll too far forward, causing users to lose their balance.

Rolling walkers equipped with weight-activated brakes are safer to use; the walker automatically stops when the user pushes down on the rear legs of the device. Some four-wheel walkers are equipped with baskets and seats that allow individuals to carry objects and sit down when tired, although sitting down requires good transfer technique and sitting balance.

ENVIRONMENTAL STRATEGIES

When older people enter a hospital or nursing facility, they are exposed to new environmental conditions such as the design of furnishings, illumination, and ground surfaces. If these conditions exceed these individuals' mobility capacity, the individuals are at risk for falls. Patients and residents with functional disabilities are especially vul-

Table 4-3.   Ambulation device inspection summary

Inspect	Examine canes and walkers for defects (e.g., worn rubber tips, defective wheels, structural problems). Replace device as indicated and/or refer all problems to physical therapy.
Inquire	Ask patients and residents about their device: Are they using their cane or walker? If not, why? Are they experiencing any problems with their cane or walker? If yes, what are the problems? Does the device improve or interfere with ambulation? Refer all problems to physical therapy.
Observe	Ask patients and residents to perform walking and transferring maneuvers with their device. Observe whether they are performing tasks correctly and safely. Is the person able to use their device properly in tight places (e.g., bathroom, bedroom) without interference? Refer all problems to physical therapy.

nerable. These individuals have a narrower adaptive range available to them to cope with the increased demands of the environment (e.g., elevated bed heights, diminished lighting, glare-producing floor surfaces). In this context, the goal of environmental interventions to reduce fall risk is twofold: 1) to identify and subsequently eliminate conditions that may interfere with mobility, and 2) to simplify or maximize individual mobility tasks by modifying the physical environment and the surrounding areas (see Chapter 5).

The most important environmental items to be assessed follow. To ensure that safe conditions are maintained, a complete and comprehensive assessment should be executed on a regular basis.

Illumination

- Are lights bright enough to compensate for reduced vision?
- Are lights glare-free?
- Are light switch plates, lamp pull cords, and switches in the bedroom and bathroom both visually and physically accessible?
- Are light switches available by the entryways of bedrooms and bathrooms (to avoid ambulating in the dark)?
- Are night-lights available in the bedroom and bathroom?

Floor surfaces

- Are floor surfaces slip-resistant and glare-free?
- Are carpeted edges secured to the floor?
- Are throw rugs slip-resistant?
- Are frequently traveled pathways in the bedroom and ward area free of low-lying (i.e., difficult to visualize) objects?

Furnishings

- Are beds low in height and stable enough to support safe, independent transfers?
- Are chairs equipped with armrests, and are they stable enough (i.e., nontippable) to support safe, independent transfers?
- Are bedside and dining room tables stable enough to support balance when leaned on?

Table 4-4. Components of policy for incident reporting

The policy clearly defines what events constitute a reportable fall (e.g., an unanticipated event, usually of sudden onset, in which the patient or resident engages in an activity that results in balance loss and a subsequent fall).

The policy clearly describes what actions to take in the event of injury and/or acute medical conditions.

The policy clearly describes fall precaution measures to follow in order to prevent recurrence.

The policy clearly outlines a step-by-step procedure to follow for completing the incident report.

The policy clearly describes a step-by-step process to follow after the incident report is completed (e.g., documenting the incident in the patient's or resident's chart; forwarding a copy of the incident report for administrative review to the medical and nursing director, safety committee, or quality assurance committee).

The policy describes a process to inform all staff involved in patient or resident care of the current policy (e.g., during orientation, during in-service education).

The policy describes a time period in which statements are updated to reflect institutional attempts to practice reasonable standards of care related to fall prevention.

Bathroom

- Are toilet grab bars available and securely fastened to the toilet or mounted on the wall?

FALL PREVENTION PROGRAMS*

Fall prevention programs have been developed by several hospitals and nursing facilities. These programs have met with varying degrees of success in fall reduction and have the following in common:

- A multidisciplinary safety committee to develop and implement an institution-wide fall prevention program.
- An in-service nursing and medical staff education program for all professionals involved in patient and resident care. Nursing education extends to staff on all three shifts.

---

*Section Two includes a comprehensive description and discussion of fall prevention programs.

- A mechanism to identify patients and residents at fall risk immediately on admission and, subsequently for each nursing shift, whenever a change of condition occurs.
- A mechanism (e.g., colored wrist identification bands, colored adhesive stickers near the bedroom door and bedside and on medical/nursing charts) for identifying at-fall-risk patients/residents.
- Assessment of patients and residents immediately after a fall.
- A formal program and policy for reporting and investigating incident reports. (The essential components of both policy and the report itself are described in Tables 4-4 and 4-5).
- Implementation of strategies to prevent falls, and follow-up to review whether the designed interventions have decreased falls on a regular basis. (These preventive strategies are presented in Table 4-6. This list is not meant to be all-inclusive, nor does it suggest that these strategies are effective. It represents those recommendations most commonly found in the literature.)
- An educational program for patients, residents, and family members that teaches the causes and prevention of falls during a stay in the hospital or nursing facility (Table 4-7).
- A discharge teaching program for patients, residents, and family members that teaches the prevention of risks of readmission (Table 4-8).
- The consistent recognition of staff (i.e., regularly given "pats on the back").

Table 4-5. Components of incident report

✍	Time and place of the fall
✍	Injuries and/or medical conditions present at the time and results of the medical examination
✍	Circumstance of the fall (patient/resident description of the event and/or eyewitness reports)
✍	Fall risk factors, both intrinsic and extrinsic, present at the time of the fall
✍	Preventive measures in place at the time of the fall, especially if the individual was at risk
✍	Immediate preventive strategies put in place to prevent additional falls
✍	Recommendations for treatment (i.e., intervention strategies) to prevent fall recurrence

- Staff are informed that their efforts have led to a reduction of falls and an enhanced level of care.

Although further research is needed, ample evidence suggests that incorporating these components into existing or newly developed fall prevention programs is beneficial in reducing fall risk.

Table 4-6. Strategies for fall prevention

Assessment

Identify fall risk on admission.

After admission, reassess risk level at regular intervals (e.g., daily, every shift, changes in medical and/or functional conditions).

Observe patient or resident mobility on a daily basis.

Monitor high-risk medications (side effects), polypharmacy.

Conduct environmental safety rounds on a regular basis (e.g., check wheelchair brakes/footrests, bed wheel brakes, bed side rail attachments, nonslip strips along the side of the bed, safety of assistive ambulation devices, condition of floor coverings, position of furnishings in bedroom, safety of bedside commodes, clutter in hallways, night-lights in bedroom, safety of footwear).

Nursing Care

Maintain regular toileting schedules (elimination rounds).

Use bedside commodes during hours of sleep.

Provide properly fitting, nonslip footwear.

Place confused patients or residents close to nurses' station for close observation.

Establish frequent nursing rounds on high-risk patients or residents.

Provide assistive ambulation.

Encourage daily exercise.

Increase nursing staff.

Environmental

Keep bed in a low position.

Keep the bed wheels locked.

Use bed half side rails to assist with safe bed transfers.

Place the call light and other objects within easy patient or resident reach.

Use bed/chair alarm systems to monitor unsafe activity.

Maintain adequate illumination in bedrooms and bathrooms.

Maintain nonslip floor surfaces.

Keep hallways clear.

Provide grab bars and toilet risers in the bathroom.

Table 4-7. Educational program for patients, residents, and family members

To reduce the risk of falls during a stay in the hospital or nursing facility:

Orient patients or residents to bedroom, unit, activities, and routines.

Orient patients or residents to staff members.

Instruct patients or residents on the proper use of equipment (e.g., electric beds, call lights, ambulation devices, wheelchairs, bathroom grab bars, bed half side rails, bedside commodes). Do not assume that individuals can figure out these things by themselves.

Teach patients or residents safe transfer techniques from bed, chairs, toilet, and wheelchair.

Instruct high-risk patients or residents to call for assistance when getting out of bed, ambulating, and toileting.

Educate family members about safety measures and fall prevention; provide instruction on how to identify risk and environmental hazards.

Provide a safety brochure that addresses important issues such as the need to wear nonslip footwear and use assistive devices whenever out of bed, the importance of calling for assistance during periods of increased risk, important side effects of medications, what to do if a fall occurs, and so forth. Material should be printed in large type for easier reading and reinforced verbally with patients or residents and family members at the time of admission.

Table 4-8. Discharge teaching program

To reduce the risk of falls and related injury at home:

Prevent the risk of down time (i.e., person is unable to arise unassisted from the floor following a fall). Provide patient or resident with a personal emergency response system (PERS). This is a button device worn by the individual as a pendant or wrist band and includes a radio transmitter connected to the person's home telephone. When the device is activated, the emergency signal goes out to a 24-hour monitoring center, which sends appropriate help (e.g., family member, neighbor, police, ambulance). The PERS can be purchased, leased, or rented. As an alternative, individuals can be taught how to rise from the floor by themselves (i.e., move themselves to a side-sitting position). They can then kneel with the support of a chair and, using the strongest knee, push themselves up into the chair.

Teach home safety. Provide the patient or resident with information about how to prevent falls in the home (see Section Two, Part B for discharge teaching sheets). In addition, patients or residents with mobility impairment should receive a home safety evaluation from physical or occupational therapists and instruction on home medical equipment required (e.g., walkers, wheelchairs, toilet and bathtub devices). Remember that equipment used in the hospital or nursing facility may not be adequate to support safe mobility in the home.

ENDNOTES

1. Lauritzen, J.B., Peterson, M.M., & Lund, B. (1993). Effect of external hip protectors on hip fractures. *Lancet, 341*, 11–13.
2. Ekman, A., Mallmin, H., Michaelsson, K., & Ljunghall, S. (1997). External hip protectors to prevent osteoporotic hip fractures. *Lancet, 350*, 563–564.
3. Hubacher, M., & Wettstein, A. (2001). Acceptance of hip protectors for hip fracture prevention in nursing homes. *Osteoporosis International, 12*, 794–799.

environmental modifications

Older adults residing in hospitals and nursing facilities differ in their functional capacity: Some have no limitations, whereas others experience partial to severe loss of function. For people with diminished physical capacity, the physical environment takes on greater significance. It can either contribute to hazardous mobility and increase the risk of falls or it can be utilized as a resource to compensate for individual mobility problems and reduce the risk of falls. For example, poor lighting increases the degree of functional visual loss and adversely affects ambulation, but it can be improved to provide a level of illumination that facilitates safe walking. Low-seated chairs without armrests can cause unsafe transfers in people with diminished muscular strength. Furniture can be made more supportive with the addition of seat cushions and armrests.

For patients and residents with decreased mobility, environmental modification can serve as a powerful adaptive strategy to promote mobility and reduce the likelihood of falling. Thus, the design of institutional environments and any subsequent adjustments must transcend appearances and be based on activity-based standards: Function must take precedence over aesthetics. Put plainly, floor surfaces and coverings, lighting, and furnishings, in structure and design, should 1) maximize or support ambulation and transferring function and 2) be aesthetically pleasing. This chapter focuses on aspects of the hospital and nursing facility environment that are most likely to contribute to unsafe mobility and that suggest corrective modification.

LIGHTING

The aspect of lighting itself is influenced by numerous factors, including illumination, location, quality, changes in intensity, access, and glare reduction.

Illumination

The proper amount of illumination in the environment is dependent on the visual needs of patients and residents. As a rule of thumb, older people require two to three times more light than do younger people to facilitate vision because of the aging-related decline in visual functioning. This is, however, a generalization. In some cases, lower levels of lighting may be more appropriate than higher levels. For instance, people with cataracts or glaucoma tend to be sensitive to bright light. For these individuals, any increase in lighting may impair their vision and increase their fall risk.

Under ideal circumstances, the control of lighting levels should rest with the individual so that he or she is able to regulate and maintain a level of illumination that is both visually comfortable and safe for mobility. Rheostatic light switches allow a person to increase or decrease illuminating levels as desired (Figure 5-1). However, patient or resident control of lighting may not always be possible, especially with individuals who have cognitive impairments or who are in wheelchairs. The best way to help determine the lighting needs of an individual is to observe the person in his or her environment and note any difficulties encountered. Correction may call for increasing, decreasing, or redistributing lighting levels.

Figure 5-1. Rheostatic light switch.

Strategic Lighting

Extra lighting may be needed in certain locations, such as the bedroom, that represent high fall risk. The path from the bedside to the bathroom may be difficult to visualize, especially at night when patients and residents may get up to go to the bathroom. In an attempt

Figure 5-2. Lighting sources that increase illumination.

to provide adequate illumination and safe passage, staff members sometimes leave the bathroom light on throughout the night. The bright bathroom light, however, may interfere with sleep or may temporarily blind the person with a sudden flooding of bright light when he or she enters the bathroom. Conversely, leaving a bright bathroom and walking into a dark bedroom can cause similar problems because older eyes readjust to lighting levels more slowly than do younger eyes.

A bedside lamp with a secure base that will not tip over, a light attached to the headboard within easy reach, or a night-light can be used to provide adequate illumination and facilitate safe ambulation (Figure 5-2). A light can be installed under the apron of a bedside table or nightstand to provide night lighting, or night-lights can be positioned close to the floor along the path leading from the bedroom to the bathroom. Motion-sensor lighting located in the bathroom is also a good solution.

Effective Lighting Sources

In addition to an adequate quantity of illumination, the quality of available lighting is important for safe ambulation. Full-spectrum fluorescent lighting is much more effective than incandescent lighting for overall illumination in the environment. Blue fluorescent light simulates natural sunlight, providing light that is spread evenly and is continuous and free of shadows. However, the best effects are produced by a bulb emitting light that is in the yellow spectrum. Halogen lamps produce light that is more like natural sunlight and freer from glare than either fluorescent or incandescent fixtures. Halogen lamps are particularly effective for task lighting, illuminating specific areas in the bedroom and bathroom. Because these lamps get quite hot, however, safety precautions should be observed.

Lighting Changes

The ability of the eye to adapt to changes in illumination decreases with age. Any sudden change in light intensity—that which occurs when a person moves from a dark to a bright area and vice versa—should be avoided because it can lead to momentary visual loss and increase the risk of falls. Perhaps the most common example involves traveling at night from a darkened bedroom into the bathroom and turning on the light. Rheostatic light switches that vary the amount of available light can ensure an even distribution of light and prevent such sudden and pronounced shifts in illumination that may occur with toggle light switches. Another alternative is to use compact fluorescent bulbs in transition areas or in rooms and areas where older people encounter dramatic changes in light levels. These bulbs take approximately 1 minute to heat to full brightness, minimizing the adjustment from darkness to light. Night-lights can be used in the bedroom and bathroom as well but are not as effective. Also, night-lights can produce frightening shadows or create an illusion of steps or edges where light and shadows meet.

Lighting Access

All environmental lighting should be physically accessible to patients and residents. Light switches should be positioned approximately 32 inches off the floor and located directly on the outside or inside of doorways to help people avoid walking across a darkened room to turn on a light (Figure 5-3). The color of the switch plates should contrast that of the wall to allow for improved visibility. If the wall and switch plate colors are identical, the switch plate should be painted in a contrasting color or adhesive tape in a contrasting color should be placed around the borders of the switch plate to enhance its visibility. A small light located within the switch or an illuminated switch plate will allow for improved visibility and access at night. Pressure-plate controls are easier to use than standard toggle switches. The pull cord that controls bedside lighting should be long enough for users to avoid excessive reaching and risk loss of balance. In addition, the pull cord should be in a contrasting color so that it can be seen easily by the older user.

Glare Reduction

Glare from sunlight shining through windows, skylights, or other light sources such as fluo-

Figure 5-3. For ease in reaching, the light switch should be located 32 inches in height from the floor.

rescent lights reflecting directly on polished waxed floors, on furnishings such as laminated tabletops, and on plastic chair seats produces discomfort or visibility glare and can impair a person's vision. Draperies or adjustable Venetian blinds can be used to block sunlight from windows. Unfortunately, they reduce the amount of available light and may not present the best solution to glare. Furthermore, horizontal and vertical blinds, with their tilting capability, cause sunlight to be deflected, creating light patterns on the floor that can be confusing visually. Polarized window glass or tinted Mylar shades can eliminate glare without loss of ambient light. Another solution is translucent light-filtering pleated shades or sheer draperies, which diffuse light and offer some degree of light and glare regulation.

Floor glare can be controlled by using carpeting or nongloss floor waxes and finishes that diffuse rather than reflect light and eliminate glare. Also, wall-mounted valances or covered lighting fixtures that conceal the source of light and spread it indirectly on the ceiling and floor serve the same purpose. Matte or dull finishes on tabletops and nonreflective material on chair seats can help prevent surface glare.

FLOOR SURFACES

Floor surfaces can be dangerous for individuals with gait and balance impairments. By identifying dangerous flooring conditions and applying some simple modifications to make floor surfaces safer, the risk of falls and injury can be reduced greatly.

Ceramic and Linoleum Surfaces

Highly polished or wet flooring can contribute to slip-related falls. In addition, highly buffed and polished flooring can cause reflected glare, the result of lighting sources shining directly on it. Glare can give floors the appearance of being wet or slick, creating a fear of falling and/or injury in some older people and leading to uncertainty or a reluctance on the part of the patient or resident to walk on the floor surface. Floor surfaces that inhibit ambulation can be viewed as a form of passive restraint, a condition resulting in restricted mobility.

Two modifications are helpful in eliminating these hazards by making bathroom and other floors skid-resistant. These modifications are 1) unglazed tile or adhesive strips and 2) antiskid acrylic coating or no-wax vinyl flooring. First, ceramic tiles and linoleum floors must be slip-resistant, particularly when wet. Unglazed tiles, which are nonslip by design, can be used in the bathroom, or slip-resistant adhesive strips can be applied to the floor next to the sink and toilet, locations that are prone to water and urine spillage (Figure 5-4). Because the purpose of adhesive strips is to help render the floor slip-resistant, it is not necessary for them to be seen. The color of the adhesive strips should match that of the floor surface to prevent easy visualization. Older people, especially those with altered

Figure 5-4. Slip-resistant adhesive strips are applied to the floor by the sink and toilet.

depth perception or dementia, may misinterpret color-contrasted floor strips, perceiving them as ground elevations or depressions that they may attempt to avoid. Individuals may try to step over the strips, thereby actually increasing their risk of falls because of alterations in gait and balance. Sheet rubber flooring in the bathroom can be used as an alternate method of slip resistance.

The second modification is to make linoleum floors slip-resistant by applying antiskid acrylic coating or by using no-wax sheet vinyl flooring. If tile and vinyl flooring are waxed, minimal buffing after waxing helps to reduce slipping and eliminates glare. Using nongloss wax as opposed to high-gloss finishes on flooring also corrects glare.

All flooring should be flush and even to prevent patients and residents from tripping on it. Doorway thresholds, such as those on the floor between the bedroom and bathroom, should be avoided or eliminated. Thresholds create a problem for older people who have poor eyesight and/or difficulty lifting their feet to clear obstacles.

Carpeting

Carpeting offers several advantages in hospital and nursing facility settings: It provides a slip-resistant surface and cushion that helps to reduce the risk of injury following a fall. In particular, indoor-outdoor carpeting in the bathroom is beneficial in that it traps water or other liquids, such as urine, that may be present, and dries quickly, thereby reducing the likelihood of slipping. As compared with vinyl flooring, a carpeted bedroom floor greatly reduces the risk of injury from a fall by providing a much softer surface on which to land.[1] Carpeting also has acoustic value in that it reduces echo resulting from shoes striking tile and linoleum flooring.

Carpeting has disadvantages as well. Older adults who use wheeled walkers and wheelchairs may experience difficulty rolling these assistive devices over carpeted surfaces, especially those that are thick. Patients and residents who push along pick-up–style walkers rather than lift up and put down the walker with each step also may experience problems with carpeting. The legs of the walker can catch on the carpet, causing an older person to lose his or her balance and fall. In addition, individuals who walk with a shuffling gait may find that thick carpeting impedes safe mobility and increases the risk of tripping.

Despite concerns about carpeting, institutions should not be discouraged from using it; when properly chosen, its advantages far outweigh any disadvantages. Uncut, low-pile carpeting is the best choice for institutional settings because this surface is least likely to interfere with walking and using walkers and wheelchairs. Deep-pile carpeting should be avoided. Aside from interfering with safe ambulation, dense carpets can cause a loss of proprioceptive feedback and balance, which are gained from the feet striking the ground. Carpet tiles are usually not recommended in institutional settings because the number of seams between the tiles creates an opportunity for liquids to seep into the underlayer. The greatest concern is that of urine seepage, the odor of which can become offensive to patients or residents, staff, and visitors alike.

Carpets made of nylon fibers provide a smooth walking surface and possess excellent strength and durability, beneficial features in areas subject to heavy traffic and soiling. The color of the carpeting should contrast with that of the walls to help older people, especially individuals with impaired depth perception, define the boundary between the floor and wall. A person's balance may be affected adversely when this distinction is not made clear. Patterns such as floral or checkered configurations, although pleasing to look at, should be avoided because they can lead to misjudgment of spatial distances. Misperception is heightened in people with a visual dysfunction, such as cataracts and poor depth perception, and dementia (i.e., patterns seem to move, leading an individual to feel increasingly confused and unbalanced). Plain, unpatterned carpeting is less confusing, both visually and intellectually. All carpeting should be checked periodically for curled edges and excessive wear in order to guard against tripping, as well.

Transitions from one type of floor surface to another must be as smooth and level as possible (i.e., no higher than ¼ inch) to accommodate wheelchairs, shuffling feet, and ambulation assistive devices. Changes in floor surfaces should be avoided in areas prone to shifts in lighting because the eyes of older adults need time to adjust to changing light levels, and these individuals may not recognize changes in surfaces in time to adjust their gait. Transitions in floor surfaces should occur only in locations where lighting is sufficient and constant.

HALLWAYS

Hallways can present an obstacle for patients and residents. Long hallways are a particular problem because they require older people with mobility problems to travel a considerable distance to reach the nurses' station, dining rooms, and so forth. As a result, patients and residents may be reluctant to walk distances, especially if they become fatigued easily, experience balance problems, or fear falling. One solution to this problem is to move the patient or resident to a bedroom that is located closer to the nurses' station and other commonly used areas. However, relocation may not be safe or easy to achieve; for example, new environments may be disorienting for people with dementia. A more realistic and perhaps better solution is to provide "rest stops," or chairs strategically placed every 20–30 feet along long hallways. These rest stops allow older individuals to rest whenever they become tired or unsteady and to continue their journey when they feel better.

Hallways and traffic lanes can become cluttered with medicine, laundry and food carts, cleaning equipment, wheelchairs, unused walkers, and poorly placed furniture, which present obstacles and interfere with safe ambulation. Clutter should be avoided as much as possible. Because many older people lose peripheral vision, they can easily bump into objects located in their path and may trip or lose balance as a result. Moreover, cluttered hallways can obstruct a person's view of handrails or access to them.

Handrail Support

In all areas used by ambulating patients and residents, handrails should be installed to provide support (e.g., enhance balance, encourage movement, allay fear of falling). Handrails are especially helpful in areas with poor footing (e.g., polished or slick flooring) or if abrasive wall finishes or coverings are present that can cut into fragile aging skin easily if walls are relied on for mobility support (i.e., hand or shoulder support) and brushed up against. Handrails are most effective for gripping if they are round rather than flat. Round handrails allow a person's thumb and forefingers to meet; flat handrails are difficult to grasp, particularly for people with arthritic hands, and are less

Figure 5-5. Handrail support should be located 2 inches from the wall and 26–36 inches in height from the floor.

effective than round handrails for maintaining support. In addition, the color of the handrails should contrast with that of the walls to promote easy visibility, should be nonslip (e.g., a wraparound cover of textured vinyl) when grasped, and should be located approximately 2 inches from the wall and 26–36 inches above the floor for easy access (Figure 5-5). Handrails that are well designed and well placed allow older people to grasp the rails and glide along them. They also allow individuals to lean on their forearms for added support.

BEDS

For patients and residents with diminished mobility skills, modification of the bed and its surrounding area can support safe mobility.

Bed Height

Bed height is defined as the distance from the floor to the tip of the mattress. Bed height is appropriate when a person is able to sit on the edge of the mattress with the knees flexed at 90° and plant both feet firmly on the floor (Figure 5-6). A bed height that is safe enough to support transfer activity can be obtained with the use of height-adjustable "hi-low" beds. Because the "hi-low" bed can be lowered to any level desired, it can provide a greater sense of security and confidence to patients and residents, which promotes independence and ease of transfers. If the height of the bed is still too great despite the use of this mechanism, a thinner mattress may be used to achieve the desired height. Because bed height may be altered routinely in order to change linens or perform routine nursing care, staff should check the height periodically to ensure that it is maintained at a level that is appropriate for the patient or resident. Also, if the beds are controlled manually with crank handles, staff should check that the handles are recessed underneath the bed at all times so that they do not constitute a tripping hazard.

Institutional bed design has changed dramatically over the past several years. Most likely, this change occurred in response to the persistent problem that falls from bed represent for hospitals and nursing facilities and to a general dissatisfaction with the type of beds available. As a result, the types of beds on the market fit various needs. Apart from a new generation of "hi-low" beds, which can be positioned at varying heights ranging from near-floor level to elevations considerably higher than standard beds,

Figure 5-6. Bed height is appropriate when the person in able to sit with the knees flexed at 90° and both feet planted firmly on the floor.

several models of fixed low–deck-height beds are available. These beds have a mattress deck height of 5½–7 inches above the level of the floor and are designed to eliminate the use of mechanical restraints for patients and residents at risk of falling from bed. The use of the "hi-low" bed can replace the common practice of placing the older person's mattress or double mattress directly on the floor to eliminate falls from bed. Although placing the mattress on the floor is effective, family members can become upset over seeing their loved one lying on the mattress, especially if the floor or carpet is not clean. In this case, families may find fixed low-height beds a better alternative. In addition, these beds are equipped with casters, which permit the bed to be moved when the floor is cleaned.

Bed Supports

Sometimes patients and residents with poor bed or walking mobility may use the footboard as an aid in transferring in and out of bed or in ambulating about the bedroom. To provide adequate support, the footboard should be easy to grasp and slip-resistant. Nonslip adhesive strips placed along the top length of the footboard prevent hands from slipping (Figure 5-7). A color-contrasted strip on the footboard can help a person to recognize it more easily, calls attention to the board itself, and helps prevent the person from bumping into the bed.

Figure 5-7. Nonslip adhesive strip is placed along the footboard to support mobility.

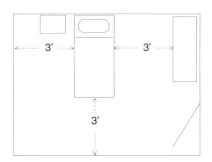

Figure 5-8. Bedroom circulation space.

In addition, an adequate amount of space between the bed and other furnishings should be created to allow for safe ambulation and transferring, particularly if walkers are used. A circulation space of at least 3 feet provides enough room for patient or resident movement with or without ambulation devices (Figure 5-8).

Mattresses

Patients and residents with poor sitting balance may be at risk for falling from bed if mattress edges sag or slouch. An overly soft mattress does not provide the support necessary for safe bed transfers, particularly if these individuals rely on hand support to accomplish them. All mattresses should be firm enough to support older adults securely when they are seated in an upright position. Mattress edges that are rolled offer individuals a good grasping surface when transferring (Figure 5-9).

Figure 5-9. Rolled mattress edge.

Bed Side Rails

Bed side rails have both disadvantages and advantages. As mentioned previously, bed side rails in the raised position can contribute to falls and physical injury. For example, patients and residents who are agile may climb over the top of the rail and become entangled in it. If they are used properly, bed side rails offer real benefits, however, providing safety and assistance in bed transfers. When positioned at least 14 inches above the top of the mattress, full-length bed side rails can help prevent people under sedation from rolling and falling out of bed unexpectedly. With one full-length bed side rail up on the opposite side of the bed, patients and residents are reminded of the side of the bed from which they should exit. However, full-length rails should not be used for individuals who are able to get out of bed. A better choice is to use half-bed side rails, which do not interfere with exiting but help prevent older adults from rolling out of bed inadvertently.

Many patients and residents are accustomed to sleeping on a wider bed surface at home, and in the hospital or nursing facility they must adjust to sleeping in a smaller bed. The standard hospital bed has several inches or, sometimes, several feet less space than what older adults are used to, increasing their risk for rolling out of bed. People with dementia or confusion may not be able to make the adjustment to a smaller bed surface, so they are at particular risk. Also, nurse call bell cords that are out of reach can cause rolling or falling out of bed because people may lose their balance while attempting to reach the call bell.

Placing a pillow or rolled blanket under the mattress edge to create a lip or "bumper" guard can be used to prevent individuals from rolling out of bed, but this intervention may lead to transfer problems when exiting beds. Some staff have adopted the practice of placing a mattress on the floor alongside the bed to prevent injuries if a fall from bed occurs. This strategy, however, may cause additional problems; for example, older people and even staff members may trip over the mattress if left in place when the bed is not occupied. In addition, staff may need to place and remove the mattress several times a day, which can lead to noncompliance with this strategy. A manufactured soft vinyl and specially designed foam floor mat (approximately 35 inches wide, 70 inches long, and 2 inches thick) has been used in some settings as an alternative to accommodate the sudden impact of a fall from bed. The mat can be walked on and left in place while direct care is provided. However, a certain amount of caution needs to be taken when floor mats are used. Patients and residents with loss of proprioception can encounter balance problems and fall risk when walking on the mat.

Figure 5-10.   Half-bed side rail is used as an assistive device.

Appropriately placed half-bed side rails can function as assistive or enabling devices, supporting people who have poor sitting and transfer balance such as those with Parkinson's disease or those who have had a stroke (Figure 5-10). Also, the rails can help older adults build confidence in their ability to safely transfer from bed, thus, reducing their fear of falling. When used as enabling devices, conventional bed side rails have some design problems. Some bed side rails are hard to grasp securely, especially for people with upper extremity dysfunction; also, bed side rails may not be secure enough to support bed transfers. As an alternative, transfer handles are available: They mount to metal bed frames, providing good stability, which allows older individuals to pull themselves up and out of bed. If bed side rails or transfer handles are used in transfers as safety devices rather than as restraints, it is a good idea to document this use in the chart. When bed side rails are not in use and are in the down position, they should recess completely underneath the bed to prevent people from climbing on the rails to enter or leave the bed.

Routine bed side rail use has long been considered standard practice in hospitals and nursing facilities. However, even half-rail use should not be ordered routinely without asking staff a few questions: "What do you hope to achieve with the use of bed side rails (e.g., will they prevent or facilitate the patient's/resident's physical and cognitive function)?" "Does the older person want you to use bed side rails?" (Patients and residents have the right to refuse bed side rails. If patients and residents cannot make their preferences known, family members should be consulted.) (See Side Rail Utilization Assessment on page 173.)

Bed Wheels

Bed wheels constitute a special hazard because they may roll or slide away during patient and resident transfers. Although all beds, including those with adequate wheel-locking systems, are unsteady to some degree, a combination swivel-and-wheel brake provides the most stability. Even when bed wheels lock properly, the bed may slide, especially if the wheels are resting on a slippery linoleum floor. To prevent sliding, the flooring can be rendered slip-resistant by placing nonslip adhesive strips or decals on the floor directly underneath the wheels (Figure 5-11). Beds that are equipped with immobilizer legs—the wheels recess when the legs are down on the floor—are an acceptable alternative to sliding bed wheels or malfunctioning locking systems (Figure 5-12).

A slippery floor surface surrounding the bed area can cause the feet of older adults to slide during bed transfers. Slippage can be prevented: Placing nonslip adhesive strips on the floor along the length

Figure 5-11. Nonslip adhesive strips placed underneath the bed wheels prevent slippage.

Figure 5-12. Bed with immobilizer legs.

Figure 5-13. Nonslip adhesive strips are placed on the floor to prevent falls.

of the bed provides the feet with a slip-resistant surface (Figure 5-13). The color of the nonslip strips should blend with the color of the floor so that people with altered depth perception do not misinterpret the strips as hazards. In addition, patients and residents should wear slip-resistant footwear when transferring in and out of bed. Some older people may not take the time to put on slippers when exiting bed. For these individuals, socks with nonslip or traction soles are a good choice.

Bed Alarm Systems

Even after instituting comprehensive bed modifications, a certain number of patients and residents remain at risk for falls. People with cognitive dysfunction (e.g., dementia, depression, delirium) are at particular risk. Cognitive losses can cause errors in judgment, such as an inability to recognize a difference between safe and hazardous bed transfers. People with neuromuscular disorders—Parkinson's disease, stroke—and poor bed mobility who fail to ask for staff assistance are also at risk. In an effort to avoid the use of mechanical or chemical restraints, some institutions use nursing assistants or family members as in-room sitters for patients and residents at risk for bed falls. In other institutions, nurses conduct hourly "bed rounds," usually at night, checking on the safety of patients and residents while in bed. Both interventions are costly because they require extra nursing staff. Bed alarm systems can be used as alternatives to in-

Table 5-1. Types of bed alarm systems

Bed and Patient- or Resident-Attached Systems

Bed and patient- or resident-attached alarms consist of a sensor unit mounted to the bed headboard and garment clip (cord), which attaches to the individual's night clothing. When the person attempts to leave his or her bed, the cord detaches from the sensor unit, sounding an alarm.

Bed-Attached Systems

Bed-attached alarms consist of a signal unit mounted on the headboard and a pressure-sensitive sensor pad or strip placed either underneath the bed linens or mattress. When the individual attempts to leave the bed, the sensor strip detects the absence of weight and sounds the alarm. Some systems are equipped with a receiver console, which can be kept at the nurses' station.

Patient- or Resident-Attached Systems

Patient- or resident-attached alarms consist of a small plastic-enclosed unit that attaches to the individual's upper leg with a fabric band. When the person attempts to leave the bed, the device shifts from the horizontal to the vertical position and sounds the alarm.

room sitters and bed rounds and help staff avoid the use of mechanical restraints to prevent bed falls. Bed alarms are designed to warn nursing staff that patients or residents who should not attempt to leave their bed unassisted are doing so.

A variety of bed alarm systems are available, some of which attach to both the bed and the patient or resident, some to the individual alone, and others to the bed alone (see Table 5-1). All systems function similarly and allow people to maintain a free-movement zone or an area adequate for normal bed activity. If the patient or resident leaves the bed and exceeds the free-movement zone, an alarm sounds in the bedroom, the nurses' station, or both, indicating that the individual is about to transfer from the bed. All systems, according to reports, are user-friendly; safe for patients and residents in that they cause no adverse effects; and easy to install, operate, and maintain. Some institutions use homemade bed alarm devices such as baby monitors or motion detectors, which alert staff to the person stirring from sleep or leaving the bed; and nurse call light cords or personal security alarms with pull cords fastened to bed clothing, which sounds an alarm when the person exits the bed. Although these devices are less costly than commercially available systems, they may not be as effective: They sometimes fail to work by not sounding an alarm or detecting bed movement and they break down easily.

Nurses in both hospital and nursing facility settings perceive bed alarms as capable of reducing the risk of falling and the need for mechanical restraints. Bed alarms, which do not require active participation by patients or residents to trigger, are preferable to nurse call systems, which demand active participation by individuals to activate. Institutions that use bed alarm systems as part of an overall fall prevention program have reduced bed falls by up to 85%.[2, 3] Without exception, concerned family members of patients and residents prefer alarm systems to the use of restraints, citing the preservation of dignity and autonomy that they offer.

The use of bed alarms should be based on a set of criteria that indicate that the patient or resident is at risk for bed falls:

- Patient or resident experiences fall(s) from bed.
- Patient or resident experiences fall(s) while ambulating in bedroom or bathroom shortly after leaving bed or is found on floor after an unwitnessed fall.
- Patient or resident demonstrates unsafe bed transfers.
- Patient or resident has a history of cognitive/communicative problems (e.g., forgets to use call bell or ask for assistance with bed transfers).
- Patient or resident has a history of nocturia (i.e., excessive urination at night).

Once a decision has been reached to use an alarm system, individual patient and resident characteristics should determine which type is the most appropriate. A number of factors may determine choice; for example, people with dementia may become confused and agitated by the use of systems that attach to their bodies. It may be better to use pressure-sensitive systems that rest on or lie underneath the mattress and out of view. Pressure-sensitive systems that have a built-in alarm time delay are useful for people who shift positions frequently during sleep. This system prevents the false alarms that can occur when people simply move on or off the pressure-sensor pads repeatedly. Some alarm systems are equipped with a prerecorded voice message (i.e., instructing the individual to remain in bed until help arrives), which activates automatically when the person leaves his or her bed. One potential problem with this type of system is that patients or residents with dementia might become increasingly confused because they don't understand the concept of hearing a voice without seeing a face.

An alarm system that attaches to the bed or to the person is also useful under certain circumstances. For example, the weight of the person can be a factor. People who weigh less than 100 pounds may not be able to apply sufficient weight to activate certain pressure-sensitive systems. In addition, antidecubiti pads added to the mattress may prevent activation with some alarm systems.

All bed alarm systems, even when appropriately selected, raise some common concerns that need to be addressed. The efficacy of any alarm system is dependent on the response time of the nursing staff. One of the leading concerns is that, by the time the alarm sounds, staff may not be able to respond quickly enough to prevent a fall, particularly if the person's bedroom is located a considerable distance from the nurses' station. Other than attempting to relocate this person to a bed closer to the nurses' station, a solution to this problem is to make it difficult for the patient or resident to get out of bed. A decubiti preventive water mattress filled to one-half capacity, placed on the bed in combination with full-length bed side rails, is effective in limiting quick bed exits even in the most agile person, and thus can provide nurses with adequate response time (Figure 5-14).

Skeptics contend that bed alarm systems are expensive both in terms of actual cost and manpower because additional nurses are needed to assist patients and residents. However, they are cost-

Decubiti
preventive
water
mattress

Full-length
bed rails

Figure 5-14. A bed with water mattress prevents decubiti, and full-length bed side rails prevent falls.

effective in that they prevent falls and they allow staff to avoid using restraints. When measured against the cost of injuries sustained from bed falls and nursing time spent in caring for people recovering from the complications of falls and restraints, the cost of bed alarms is worthwhile. Most devices can be billed to diagnosis-related groups and to other third-party payers by charging a daily monitoring fee or budgeting the expense under the category "capital equipment." In addition, questions may be posed concerning legal liability and bed alarm use. Despite the use of these systems, the risk of bed falls and injuries continues. Although not challenged by the courts, hospitals and nursing facilities would do well to assume a defensive position in order to protect themselves. Assuming such a position would entail documenting the use of bed alarm devices in patients' or residents' charts as well as recording the rationale. Also, the risks and benefits of alarm systems should be explained to patients and residents, if competent, and family members; written consent should be obtained as well.

Legislation eliminating the use of mechanical restraints has contributed to a proliferation of bed alarm device manufacturers. The result is healthy but confusing: Although new and improved devices are introduced routinely, the variety of choices makes it difficult to know which product to select. Bed alarm systems should meet a basic set of criteria:

- The system emits a distinctive alarm that is loud enough to be heard at the nurses' station and other locations.
- The system emits a silent alarm in the patient's or resident's bedroom and emits a loud alarm at the nurses' station so that sleeping patients or residents are not aroused by the alarm.
- The system does not interfere with patient or resident care.
- The system is easy to use and maintain by staff.
- The system is durable; warranty and service contracts are included.
- The system has performed reliably and users, both nursing staff and patients or residents, are satisfied with the product. The customer should request a list of clients.

When purchasing the system, staff should ask the manufacturer whether its devices meet these standards.

SEATING

Modification of chairs can be used to support independent and safe transfers in older adults with diminished transfer skill. Before seating can be modified, however, knowledge of seating standards is essential.

Seating Criteria

The criteria for proper seating in hospitals and nursing facilities is governed by one simple rule: Proper seating should meet the seating needs of patients and residents. To this end, chairs should assist in and not impede self-initiated transfers and provide comfort. Several methods are available to assess proper seating. Perhaps the most common is to select chairs that match the anthropometric, or body, measurements of older adults. For example:

- Seat height (Figure 5-15) is obtained by measuring a person's lower leg length, the distance from the foot on the floor to the knee or popliteal area behind the knee—generally 15–17 inches.
- Seat depth (Figure 5-16) is obtained by measuring upper leg length, the distance from the plane of the back to the popliteal area—generally 16–20 inches.
- Seat width (Figure 5-17) is obtained by measuring the distance across the widest point of the person's hips or thighs—generally

16" to 20"

15" to 17"

Figure 5-15. Seat height is appropriate when it is placed 15–17 inches from the floor.

Figure 5-16. Seat depth is appropriate when it is located 16–20 inches from the popliteal area to the buttocks.

Figure 5-17. Seat width is appropriate when it is at least 18 inches wide.

14–16 inches—and adding another 2 inches (i.e., 1 inch on each side of the hip) to prevent the body from rubbing or resting against the side of the chair.

- The height of the armrest from the seat is generally 7–7½ inches.
- The length of the armrest is generally 18–20 inches.
- The seat slope, or angle of the backrest, is generally 7–10 inches.
- The height of the backrest from the seat is generally 17 inches or higher.

Anthropometric seating criteria are useful for purchasing chairs in quantity, which is a common practice for most institutions because of the economic advantages offered. Appropriate seating requires more than simply selecting a chair or sofa that is anthropometrically correct, however. Even if these criteria are met, a person may experience problems with seating mobility. Therefore, the best method of assessing optimal seating is to observe the person actually using chairs in the environment to determine whether any difficulty is experienced. The individual performing the assessment must take into account the variability of individual anthropometric indices and the effects of different disease conditions as they affect chair mobility. The assessor must 1) watch the person sit down and rise from the chair and check that the task is performed safely and independently, and 2) ask whether the seat is comfortable when the person is seated.

Seating Height

Seat height, or the distance between the floor and the front edge of the chair, is critical to mobility. If the seat height is too low or too high, it can interfere with safe transfers. Seats that are too low require the body to move a great distance between sitting and standing positions: Greater knee flexion and leg muscle strength is necessary to initiate the upward thrust required to rise as well as support the downward motion needed to sit. This extra effort is especially hard on people whose range of motion in the knees and hips is limited and whose muscle strength is reduced. Conversely, it is much easier to transfer on and off higher level seats. High-level seating requires the body to exert less joint flexion and muscle strength for both transfer functions.

In an effort to compensate for low-level seating, people usually add either cushions or a pillow to the seat or select a higher chair on which to sit. However, compensation can be problematic. If the feet do not rest flat on the floor, the person is forced to slide from the seat to reach the floor when attempting to stand and to climb onto the seat when attempting to sit. Both movements can compromise safety. If loss of balance occurs, the person risks a fall. Seat height is appropriate when it allows the patient or resident to sit with both feet planted firmly on the floor and the knees flexed at 90° (Figure 5-18). The front of the seat should be low enough to allow for a small space between the thighs and seat (Figure 5-19). The ability of the person to pass the flat of the hand freely underneath the seated person's thigh and edge of the seat provides a good index of the space that is required between the seat and the body.

Figure 5-18. Seat height is appropriate when the person is able to sit with the knees flexed at 90° and both feet are planted firmly on the floor.

Low-level seating can be altered by providing patients and residents with chair seat heights that are functionally suited to the individual. If these heights are not available, a seating cushion can be added to the existing chair. Its width, or thickness, should be determined by how much height is needed to achieve independent mobility.

Leg Space

To facilitate rising from a chair, the provision of a kick space below a seat is essential (Figure 5-20). Proper kick space allows the person to slide one foot underneath the chair and one foot forward to obtain the leverage necessary for the lower extremities to exert maximum thrust upward. Cross-bars or cross-rails on chair legs, used to provide structural support, may interfere with rising if they are posi-

Figure 5-19. Front seat space.

Figure 5-20. Leg kick space.

tioned too low or too far forward on the chair (Figure 5-21). Cross-bars or cross-rails should be positioned high enough or set back far enough to ensure they do not interfere with the biomechanics of rising (Figure 5-22). The presence of armrests or seats that are some-what higher may compensate for poorly positioned cross-rails.

Armrests

All chairs used by older people should be equipped with armrests. Older people, much more than younger people, depend on armrests for assistance in propelling the body weight forward and maintaining balance when standing. The support offered by armrests while rising

Figure 5-21. Cross-bars positioned too far forward or too low can interfere with safe rising from a seated position.

Figure 5-22. Appropriately positioned cross-bars.

Figure 5-23. Nonsupportive armrest positions. (Left) Too low; (right) set back too far.

is additionally advantageous because it helps reduce pressure on the knee joints. Armrests also play a supportive role in helping a person to sit. A point is reached, particularly for individuals with decreased strength in the lower extremities or limited range of motion in the knee, when older adults' leg muscles and knee flexion no longer function effectively to help them sit down easily. As a result, they drop their body weight onto a seat. Armrests help arrest this quick, downward thrust of the body by assisting in its gradual descent.

Armrests that are too low, too high, or set too far back may inhibit both rising from the chair and sitting in it. Low-level armrests force a person to lean forward when rising and thus threaten balance. Armrests that are too high or set too far back cannot provide a sufficient angle of leverage for the upper extremities when rising from a seat (Figure 5-23). To achieve optimal function in providing assistance, armrests should be of the correct height, positioned horizontally 7–7½ inches above the seat (Figure 5-24). They should extend at least to the seat's edge or, ideally, 1–2 inches beyond the front edge (Figure 5-25). This position allows for maximum leverage when rising because it enables individuals to engage their stronger lower body muscles in the task of rising to a standing

Figure 5-24. Appropriate armrest height.

Figure 5-25. Appropriate armrest length.

Figure 5-26. Armrest support during transfer activities.

position, and continues to provide support until stability in standing is achieved (Figure 5-26). In addition, armrests should be nonslip, easy to grasp, and sloped slightly, more to the back than to the front, for maximum comfort.

Figure 5-27. Chair seat or backrest angles.

Seat Depth and Backrest Angle

In general, the deeper the seat (i.e., the distance measured from the popliteal area to the buttocks), the greater the effort required for the person to move the body forward to the edge of the seat to rise. In addition to length, seat depth is affected by the angle of the backrest. The greater the angle or slant, the deeper the seat depth and the greater the distance a person must negotiate to pull him- or herself up (Figure 5-27).

The backrest or slope should always be considered in relation to the ability of the person to rise independently and should support the lower back. If the seat is too deep or the angle of the backrest is

Figure 5-28. Appropriate seating
cushion.

Figure 5-29. Appropriate angle for a
seat slope.

too great, a seating cushion placed along the length of the backrest usually can correct the deficiency (Figure 5-28).

To facilitate rising from a chair, the seat should slope gently backward at an angle of no more than 1 inch from the front edge of the seat to its back edge (Figure 5-29). Seating that angles too far backward may present problems with rising because the person's knees will be positioned at a higher level than the buttocks (Figure 5-30). A seating angle that is tilted too far forward places the person's knees at a level that is lower than that of the buttocks and contributes to a slouched sitting position, which encourages sliding out of the chair (Figure 5-31). A wedge cushion can correct both problems

Figure 5-30. Inappropriate backward
seating angle.

Figure 5-31. Inappropriate forward
seating angle.

Figure 5-32. Appropriate wedged cushion.

Figure 5-33. Appropriate curved seat edge.

(Figure 5-32). The wider part of the cushion should be positioned either in front of the seat to prevent sliding or at the back to assist people who experience difficulty in rising from their seat. In addition, the front edge of the seat should curve gently to avoid placing pressure on the back of the person's knees (Figure 5-33), which restricts blood flow and causes the development of leg swelling or phlebitis.

Seating Cushions

Cushions on chairs should provide comfort and absorb the impact caused by a person sitting in a seat, but they should not be too soft. People tend to sink into overly soft cushions, making it difficult to get out of them (Figure 5-34). Moreover, overly soft cushions reduce effective seat height because they are compressed by the seated person, thus lowering the seat. As such, it is difficult to rise in one fluid motion. Also, overly soft cushions prevent people from shifting their buttocks, a natural protective motion that helps individuals avoid developing decubiti.

Figure 5-34. Inappropriate seat cushion (too soft).

The best type of seating cushions for chairs is the one that is relatively flat and firm, has some resilience, and does not "bottom out" when a person sits on it. A suitable cushion should give way when a fist is pressed firmly into it, yet resist if further pressure is applied. A cushion consisting of latex material provides pliancy sufficient for comfort and firmness, without excessive compression. Foam cushions should be avoided because they lose resilience over time and tend to bottom out. The color of the seat cushion should contrast that of the chair so that it can be seen during seating. To prevent sliding, the seat covering should be manufactured of a slip-resistant material.

Seating Stability

The stability of a chair is crucial to a person's safety. If, during the act of transferring, the chair tips forward, sideways, or backward, the risk of loss of balance and falling is increased greatly. Chairs with a seat edge that overhangs the position of the legs should be avoided. The design can cause the chair to tip forward when a person moves to its front edge or sits on the edge rather than in the middle of the seat (Figure 5-35). Casters or metal tips attached to the ends of the chair legs can be dangerous, especially on slick linoleum flooring. The weight of the body can cause chairs that are equipped with these devices to slide when the person sits, rises, or leans on the chair for balance support. Dining room chairs, in particular, can be precarious. Although dining

Figure 5-35. Inappropriate elongated seat cushion.

chairs must pull away easily from the table, casters are too unstable for most frail older people to use safely. In general, casters and metal tips should be removed. As an alternative, chairs can be placed up against the wall, which prevents them from sliding away during transfers.

Chairs are most stable when the chair legs are straight, positioned well forward of the seat's leading edge but not so splayed as to invite tripping, and the edge of the seat does not extend too far forward beyond the chair legs. In addition, some individuals with balance problems use chair backrests for mobility support. Thus, back-

Figure 5-36. Appropriate back-rest height.

Figure 5-37. A wedge cushion that slants backward prevents independent rising.

rests should be placed high enough on the chair in order to provide adequate support. In general, a height of approximately 32 inches, the distance from the floor to the top of the backrest, is sufficient for this purpose (Figure 5-36). The backrest must be nonslip for safe grasping: A nonslip adhesive strip placed along the backrest prevents slipping. A good test of a chair's stability is for a staff member to grasp and lean into the chair and slide and tilt it forward, backward, and sideways.

Seating Alternatives to Restraints

Patients and residents who experience poor mobility and remain at fall risk, despite adaptation of existing chairs, may benefit from one of several different types of seats. A deep-seated, soft-cushioned lounge chair or recliner with a seat that slants downward toward the back; a wedge cushion, the widest part of which is placed toward the front of the seat (Figure 5-37); or a beanbag chair filled with Styrofoam pellets may be alternatives to mechanical restraints. These furnishings work by keeping an individual's buttocks at a level that is lower than that of the knees, making it exceedingly difficult for the person to rise. Their purpose is to prevent the person who cannot ambulate safely from getting up independently or from sliding off of a seat. Caution is advised because this seating position places increased pressure on the buttocks, particularly on the buttocks of thin individuals, placing them at risk for developing decubiti. Although these seats are considered by some critics to be restraints because they prevent independent movement, they can help people avoid many of the harmful effects associated with mechanical restraints (see Chapter Six).

If these seating choices are unsuitable, a chair alarm system may serve as an option. A chair alarm system is a battery-powered, portable device that consists of either a cord that attaches to the person's gown or a pressure-sensitive pad that rests on the seat or against the backrest. When a patient or resident slides to the edge of the chair or attempts to stand, the device sounds an alarm that alerts the nursing staff. The indications for a chair alarm are as follows:

- Patient or resident experiences fall(s) from a chair or wheelchair
- Patient or resident experiences fall(s) while ambulating (shortly after rising from the chair) or is found on the floor next to the chair or wheelchair (unwitnessed fall)
- Patient or resident demonstrates unsafe chair/wheelchair transfers

Chair alarms are effective, but only to a point. By the time a nurse comes to assist a patient or resident, the person already may be standing or he or she may be lying on the floor. Placing pressure-sensitive pads against the chair backrest and keeping the length of clothing-attached cords short helps staff detect early departure from chairs. In order to be heard by staff, chair alarms are generally loud, which can have a negative impact on patients and residents (e.g., the loud sounds may frighten them) and lead to a fear of leaving the chair.

BATHROOM

For older adults with poor walking and transferring balance, bathrooms can be especially hazardous places. Modifications of the existing bathroom can help to support safe mobility and reduce the risk of falls and injury.

Fixture Support

Patients and residents with balance dysfunction and people who are unable to use their walkers in the bathroom because of space limitations often resort to the use of sink tops, towel bars, and wall surfaces

Figure 5-38. Bathroom grab rails.

Figure 5-39. Nonslip adhesive strips placed on a sink.

for support. These structured are poor alternatives and may contribute to falls, particularly if the individual's hand slips. Moreover, towel bars are often located too high on the wall to provide adequate support. Several modifications to eliminate this hazard are available: A grab bar placed horizontally in place of the towel bar or a grab rail that runs around the perimeter of the bathroom wall can be used to provide balance support (Figure 5-38).

The color of the grab bars should contrast that of the wall for visibility, be slip-resistant (vinyl coating offers a better gripping surface than do standard metal bars), and should be positioned no more than 1½ inches from the wall to keep a person's arm from slipping between the bar and the wall. It is important that grab bars be attached securely to wall studs so that they do not give way easily. A wide variety of grab bar lengths and angles are available, which allows health care providers to tailor grab bars to specific patient and resident needs.

Nonslip adhesive strips placed along sink tops prevent hands from sliding (Figure 5-39). The color of strips should be similar to that of the sink top to eliminate visual confusion. In addition, grab bars can be mounted on the face of vanity tops to provide an additional support surface.

Toilets

Toilets that are low in height often cause problems in transferring. To circumvent such problems, corrective modifications should be made, which can include raised toilet seats and grab bars. Raised toilet seats are available in two types: fixed and adjustable height. Several sizes of fixed-height toilet seats should be available to accommodate individual needs. It is advised that raised toilet seats be constructed of materials that are sturdy enough to provide support. The seats themselves should be made of soft vinyl or plastic to provide patients or residents with an absorptive cushion. An absorptive cushion reduces the risk of pelvic or hip fracture in people who have a tendency to drop onto the toilet seat. The color of the toilet seat should contrast that of the toilet tank and bowl and surrounding area to facilitate individual's proper seating placement, particularly in people who depend on visual cueing. Contrasting the color of bathroom walls with that of the toilet can help people to visualize the toilet as well.

The installation of grab bars on the wall next to and behind the toilet or a double armrest grab bar system, commonly referred to as a toilet safety frame, that attaches to the toilet can be used by patients and residents to maintain their balance during toileting transfers. The type and height placement of grab bars mounted to the wall depends on the individual, his or her disability, and the surrounding environment. For example, people with hemiplegia find it difficult to use grab bars placed on their dysfunctional side, people of short stature or limited reach find grab bars placed at heights that are convenient for the "average person" unsatisfactory because they are beyond their reach, and people in wheelchairs experience transfer problems with conventional grab bars and find wall-mounted "swing-up" or "hinged-arm" grab bars easier to use. (This type of grab bar folds flat against the wall directly behind the toilet when not in use and can be moved to the horizontal position when in use.)

An alternative to wall-mounted grab bars is the toilet safety frame, or double armrest system (Figure 5-40). Many older people find this grab bar easier to use because the maximum amount of force exerted during transfers is completed in a straight downward movement of the arms, which provides optimum transferring support. Conversely, wall-mounted grab bars provide less support because, when transferring, the person must reach to the side and bend forward in order to

Figure 5-40. Armrest toilet riser.

grab the bar. As a result, the direct benefit of a downward thrust offered by the double armrest system is lost. The double armrest system is convenient for staff because it is easy to attach and can be readily adjusted for an individual patient or resident. As a cautionary measure, nonslip adhesive strips in a noncontrasting color should be placed on the floor in front of the toilet to prevent the person's feet from slipping during transfers. Nurse call alarms located in the bathroom and toilet paper holders must be accessible to guard against falls from the toilet.

Patients and residents who are unable to toilet autonomously may be able to maintain independence by using a bedside commode. Beside commodes that are height adjustable for individual variation and fitted with armrest support to aid safe transfers should be chosen. Commodes that are equipped with wheels should be avoided because they can roll away easily during transfers.

TABLES AND NIGHTSTANDS

Many patients and residents with balance disorders use the edge of tabletops and nightstands for transferring and walking support. If

Figure 5-41. Pedestal table.

these furnishings are unstable or the tops are slippery when grasped, they may fail to provide balance support. Furnishings that are not supportive can cause individuals to develop a fear of falling as well. It is best to avoid pedestal-style tables, which tend to tip over easily when a person's weight is applied to the edge (Figure 5-41). Nightstands that are used to assist with bed transfers may slide away, particularly if they are equipped with wheels or metal casters. Over-the-bed tables are similarly dangerous.

All tables and nightstands in the institutional environment should be stable when leaned on or grasped. They should have nonslip surfaces. Stability can be achieved by selecting tables with four legs that are free of wheels or casters and have a slip-resistant matte surface that promotes grasping. Tabletops with a contrasting border help patients and residents identify the boundary of the table, thus promoting proper hand placement and support and averting "bumping into" accidents. Table edges that are rounded or bull nosed prevent bumping injuries that result from contact with sharp edges. Dining tables with spill-free edges, which restrain spilled liquids, are useful because they guard against wet floors and slippage. Dining room tables and chairs should work together: The arms of the chairs and wheelchairs should fit under the table to allow older people to move in as close as possible for dining and to avoid fluid spillage. To accommodate wheelchairs, tables must be approximately 34 inches high. Because the height may be exclusively for people dining in regular chairs, tables with adjustable height bases to accommodate both populations should be purchased. In addition, the position of tables and nightstands in the institutional environment should not obstruct ambulation.

STORAGE AREAS

All closets and dressers used by patients and residents must be accessible without the need for excessive reaching and bending. Frequently used items such as day and night wear and footwear should be placed on shelves or in drawers that lie between the person's eye and waist levels. This height accommodates the functional reach of most older people, thus minimizing the risk of balance loss.

ENDNOTES

1. Healey, F. (1994). Does flooring type affect risk of injury in older inpatients? *Nursing Times*, *90*, 40–41.
2. Heslin, K., Towers, J., Lecki, C., et al. (1992). Managing falls: Identifying population-specific risk factors and preventative strategies. In S.G. Funk, E.M. Tornquist, M.T. Champage, & R.A. Wiese (Eds.), *Key aspects of elder care: Managing falls, incontinence, and cognitive impairment* (pp. 70–80). New York: Springer.
3. Widder, B. (1985). A new device to decrease falls. *Geriatric Nursing*, *6*, 287–288.

chapter six

reducing mechanical
and chemical restraints

Until the 1990s, the sight of an old, frail person being restrained to a bed or chair was a familiar scene in hospitals and nursing facilities throughout the United States. Anywhere from 25% to 85% of older adults—more than half a million individuals—in these institutions were placed in mechanical restraints each day.[1] Concern about their lack of effectiveness, safety, and serious consequences have been established in the U.S. health care community and among sensitive laypeople. As a result, a nationwide effort has been under way for a number of years to reduce and, eventually, eliminate the use of restraints as a fall prevention measure. The impetus stems from consumer advocates, health professionals, and government regulators who are concerned about the negative effects of restraints and lack of effectiveness of restraints in preventing falls. As a result, policies aimed at the elimination of mechanical restraints have been developed. The most prominent policy is the Omnibus Budget Reconciliation Act (OBRA) of 1989 (PL 101-239).[2] OBRA represents a legislative concern about the quality of care in nursing facilities in general and the widespread use of restraints in particular. Implemented in 1990, one of OBRA's strongest mandates was that nursing facilities examine their use of mechanical restraints and begin to find alternatives. As a consequence of OBRA regulations, the use of restraints in nursing facilities has declined dramatically, from a prevalence rate of 41% in 1988 to a level at the beginning of the 21st century of just under 20%. The movement to reduce restraints has affected acute care hospitals as well. The Joint Commission on Accreditation of Healthcare Organizations (JCAHO) has put into place restraint-reduction initiatives for hospitals modeled after OBRA.

RATIONALE

The reasons for the use of mechanical restraints in hospitals and nursing facilities are often multifactorial, encompassing both patient and resident (host-related) and institutional factors:[3]

Patient/resident-related factors

- Prevent falls and related injury
- Decrease fall risk resulting from mobility problems, unsafe wandering, confusion, or agitated behaviors
- Correct seating alignment
- Prevent unsafe wandering
- Prevent interference with medical treatment

Institutional factors

- Frail patients and residents are at risk for falls, injury, or both if not restrained
- Inadequate staffing requires the use of restraints
- Institutions have a "moral duty" to protect patients and residents
- Failure to restrain places employees and the facility at legal risk
- Restraints allow nurses to provide efficient and timely care
- Families request and demand "risk-free" care, which includes restraint use
- Few alternatives to restraints exist

Although restraints are designed to protect patients and residents from falls and harm, they are not the best choice, nor do they represent the best solution, except possibly under extreme circumstances. As mentioned in the list, all of the firmly entrenched beliefs that support their continued use are based on myth because no documented evidence exists that restraints are effective in accomplishing the purposes for which they are used. Many studies conclude that restraints seldom eliminate the risk of injury from falls but that, conversely, they can precipitate or exacerbate the problem. Most researchers concur that people in restraints are subject to the same or added fall risk as are individuals without restraints. Among facilities that do or do not use restraints, little difference exists in the extent of fall occurrences.[4] Moreover, facilities that do restrain experience a higher incidence of serious injury following falls.[5] When restraints are removed there may be an increase in the number of falls but not in the number that result in significant injury.

Some nurses continue to believe that rendering care to patients and residents is easier and more efficient when restraints are used. Although it may appear that providing daily care to people with mobility problems is achieved more quickly when they are restrained, this strategy is ineffective. People in restraints rapidly develop immobility and associated morbidity, which creates greater dependency and need for custodial care from the staff and heightens the risk of falls. Aside from concerns about effectiveness, the use of restraints to "protect and safeguard" patients and residents is suspect. Although restraints have been applied in some instances for protective reasons (e.g., to prevent falls in people who are confused and wander when an immediate and clear threat of injury exists), the risks associated with restraints outweigh the benefits. The arguments supporting restraint use in protecting patients and residents at risk for immediate harm are questionable because alternatives have been successfully used that serve the same purpose and do not subject them to harm.

Rather than protecting older adults, restraints place them at risk for numerous detrimental physical and psychological consequences. Restraints that are too restrictive or applied too tightly can cause circulatory obstruction of the lower extremities, edema, skin abrasions, respiratory difficulties, and unintentional death by strangulation. Hospital patients who are restrained have twice the length of institutional stay of those who are free from restraints; they are also more likely to be transferred to nursing facilities for care and are at higher risk for early death. Much of the resulting mortality is the consequence of restraint use and its concomitant immobility.

The psychological consequences of restraints are many and help refute any beliefs that older people are not bothered by their use. Often, application triggers one of several emotional reactions: People feel either fear and a sense of panic, which can result in belligerent behavior, or a sense of humiliation and abandonment, which can result in aggressive behavior, a loss of self-image, depression, withdrawal, or low social functioning. In addition, self-esteem decreases because, typically, others view individuals who are in restraints as disturbed, dangerous, or mentally incompetent, which can be demoralizing. Moreover, when older adults are not informed about the decision to apply restraints or are not allowed to either accept or refuse their use, they are denied their right of self-determination. This violation of personal rights constitutes a restriction of an individual's autonomy, including the freedom to make choices about engaging in activities. When a person is restrained and denied the ability to get up, sit down, or walk about with undue interference, his or her quality of life and psychological well-being are impaired.

Health care professionals are not immune from the effects of restraints. Nurses, who are often responsible for initiating restraint orders in hospitals and nursing facilities, struggle with the burden brought on by this decision. On the one hand, they feel a professional duty to protect and safeguard people who are at risk for falls. This obligation is often heightened when nursing allocations are scarce and monitoring of problematic individuals is difficult. To avoid the risk of legal sanctions, some nurses feel that they have no alternative but to apply restraints. On the other hand, nurses find the act of restraining older people stressful and emotionally taxing, often provoking in themselves anxiety, dissatisfaction, and guilt. They recognize that restraints deprive individuals of their autonomy and dignity, and they sympathize with them, conceding that they themselves would not want to be placed in a similar position.

Although nurses perceive themselves as less vulnerable to legal sanctions if restraints are used, particularly in the event of injury, the fear of legal liability is ill founded. Despite the fact that lawsuits for damages resulting from falls are relatively common, few have been successful against facilities and their employees solely based on the failure to restrain. In cases involving injury to people without restraints, a preponderance of other factors usually constitutes negligence, including improper assessment and documentation of the patient's or resident's condition, failure to assess and monitor the person at risk for falls, and failure to respond to falls and injury in a timely manner. Rather, the use of restraints may increase the risk of litigation. Lawsuits involving the improper application of restraints that results in patient and resident injury (e.g., falling out of a bed or chair either with restraints intact or removed by the person) have been successful. In addition, facilities and staff may be held liable when restraints are used for convenience, for example, during staffing shortages.

Family members are also affected by restraint decisions and react in various ways to finding their relative restrained. Some express dismay at the sight of a relative in restraints and demand their removal, even if the action places the person at fall risk. Others, although not accepting of the practice, come to accept restraints as a necessary evil, believing that they will keep their relative from being injured in a fall. This notion is reinforced when family members are not informed by staff of the harmful effects of restraints and of the available alternatives for safeguarding their relative.

Much of the justification for using mechanical and chemical restraints is based on the misapprehension that no alternatives are available. Many hospitals and nursing facilities in the United States have deliberately reduced restraint use without experiencing a concomitant rise in serious injury. Such facilities have adopted a policy of nonrestraint use that is employed commonly in several European countries. These countries place greater emphasis on structuring the physical environment and the activities of patients and residents in such a way that restraints are rarely, if ever, needed or used.

MANAGEMENT

The challenge for health care professionals in hospitals and nursing facilities is reducing the use of mechanical and chemical restraints while decreasing the risk of falls. To achieve this objective, hospital and nursing facility staff can take a number of steps within their individual facilities:

Step 1

Examine current restraint practices, the attitudes of employees toward their use, and institutional policies that govern the use of mechanical and chemical restraints. The intent of this exercise is to determine the prevalence of restraint use; the availability, utilization, and effectiveness of restraint alternatives; and whether policies are viable and provide staff with appropriate direction in the use of restraints. Inquire about the following:

- To what extent are restraints used?
- Under what circumstances or conditions are restraints ordered and why?

- Are restraints the first or last choice in treatment?
- Are restraints effective in controlling the risk of falls?
- Are restraints used continuously, intermittently, or on a short-term basis? Under what conditions?
- Are patients and residents (if able) and family members consulted on the need for restraints and given the right of refusal?
- If either party refuses the use of restraints, what procedures are in place to ensure the patient's or resident's safety?
- Are individuals who are restrained observed or monitored for nutritional or toileting needs and adverse effects? How often? By whom?
- If individuals experience adverse effects, are restraints discontinued? If not, why? If so, what forms of management are used to replace restraints?
- Are restraint alternatives ever considered as an initial choice of treatment? Under what circumstances?
- What types of alternative treatments are available? Are they effective in controlling the problem indicated? If not, why?
- Are institutional policies clear as to the types of conditions or situations in which restraints can and cannot be used; the types of restraint alternatives available; the assessment procedure for restraint use and discontinuation; and who has the responsibility of ordering, monitoring, and documenting restraint and nonrestraint use?
- Are institutional policies updated periodically? Are staff members aware of the content in policy statements?

Step 2

Establish an ongoing program of in-service education aimed at assessing restraints (see Table 6-1) and assessing and managing the problems (e.g., dysmobility, falls, confusion, wandering, poor sitting posture) that are cited commonly as indications for restraints. These problems should not be viewed as end-stage processes but as signs of an underlying medical or environmental condition. Ordering a restraint as initial treatment is inappropriate; rather, these problems should trigger further investigation and treatment aimed at eliminating the underlying conditions responsible. If the problem persists, alternatives to the use of restraints should be explored (see Table 6-2). Restraints, if necessary, should be considered only as a

Table 6-1. Content for educational in-service training on restraints

I. **Overview of restraints**
   A. Prevalence
   B. Reasons for restraints
      1. Avoidance of falls
      2. Control of wandering behavior
      3. Control of agitation/behavioral problems
      4. Correction of seating/positioning problems
   C. Ineffectiveness of restraints in managing patient or resident safety

II. **Adverse effects of restraints**
   A. Physiological consequences
   B. Loss of autonomy
   C. Loss of dignity
   D. Agitation/depression
   E. Family and staff discomfort

III. **Legal**
   A. Current OBRA and JCAHO regulations concerning restraint use
   B. Institutional policies regarding restraints
   C. Staff liability issues

IV. **Restraint alternatives**
   A. Assessment
      1. Identify causes of fall risk
      2. Identify causes of wandering
      3. Identify causes of agitation/behavioral problems
      4. Identify causes of seating problems
   B. Nonrestraint management
      1. Modify underlying problems discovered
         a. Fall risk
         b. Wandering
         c. Agitation/behavioral manifestations
         d. Poor seating
      2. Review available restraint alternatives
         a. Approaches/methods to support seating
         b. Approaches/methods to guard against falls
         c. Approaches/methods to permit safe wandering
         d. Approaches/methods to manage behavioral manifestations
         e. Approaches/methods to support mobility

Table 6-2.   Alternatives to restraints

Caregiving
   Additional nursing supervision/observation of activities
   Assistance of family members/volunteers
      (companionship, supervision of activities)
   Daily ambulation, structured activities
   Exercise; gait/balance training
   Instruction on safe chair/wheelchair transfers
   Maintain regular toileting schedule
   Evaluate adverse medication affects
   Correct sensory deficits
      (e.g., eyeglasses, hearing aids)
   Provide safety when patient or resident judgment is impaired
Environmental
   Orient patient/resident to environment
   Arrange for patient/resident to be near nursing station
   Provide adequate lighting, night lights
   Maintain obstacle-free environment
   Provide ambulation devices
   Employ strategic seating
   Make available a variety of seating options
      (different heights, seat angles)
   Provide alternative seating
      (wedge cushions, seating props, slanting chairs, beanbag chairs)
   Provide nonslip floor surfaces
   Supply/encourage appropriate footwear
   Provide bed and chair alarms, accessible call buttons
   Lower bed height, mattress on floor
   Remove bed wheels
   Provide accessible call light
   Avoid full-length bed side rails
   Use half-bed side rails to support transfers ("enablers")
   Provide commode at bedside
   Provide perimeter alarms, safe wandering areas
   Provide Merry Walker
      (designed walker that permits independent ambulation for individuals
      with dementia or confusion)

temporary measure to be used under extreme emergency conditions or as a last resort when the advantages to the patient or resident clearly outweigh the disadvantages. To this end, attention to staff education regarding selection of appropriate restraints and their proper application is warranted. In general, the restraint chosen should be the one that is the least restrictive and safest. Both the patient or resident and the restraint should be checked frequently.

Step 3

Hospitals and nursing facilities should develop and implement restraint-reduction policies. The purpose of these policies is to provide staff with step-by-step guidelines related to mechanical restraint decisions and care for patients and residents. These documents also can serve as defense against potential legal liability because they illustrate an attempt by the institution and staff to practice reasonable standards of restraint practice. The policy statement should be clear and simple to follow and should address the following points specifically:

- Define what a mechanical restraint is and describe the types of restraining devices available.
- Define and categorize the types of situations in which restraints may or may not be used.
- Define the assessment procedure for the application and discontinuation of restraints.
- Define who has the responsibility for ordering and discontinuing restraints.
- Define the procedure and staff responsibilities for documenting restraint use.
- Define the procedure for monitoring restraint use.
- Define the types of circumstances under which restraint alternatives should be considered.
- Define the types of restraint alternatives available.
- Define the procedure to follow when patients and residents or family members refuse restraints.
- Define a procedure for ensuring that all staff are aware of the institution's policy and that the contents of the policy are updated periodically.

Reducing mechanical restraints may be difficult to achieve in all instances, and perhaps more so in the acute care hospital than in the nursing facility setting. It is important to recognize that, with respect to fall-prevention efforts, "good" care consists of helping patients and residents to achieve maximum independence while attempting to reduce the likelihood of falls. It is clear that there are few justifications for the use of mechanical restraints and that restraints are more likely to cause falls than prevent them.

Health care providers also must be cognizant of chemical restraints—the misuse of psychoactive medications—and eliminate this practice. The most common categories of psychoactive medications include antipsychotics (i.e., neuroleptics or major tranquilizers), anxiolytics (i.e., antianxiety or minor tranquilizers), sedatives and hypnotics (i.e., sleep inducers), and antidepressants. Often, these drugs are prescribed to control mood, mental status, or behaviors—acute confusional states, agitated or violent behaviors, anxiety, depressive states, wandering—that place patients and residents at risk for falls or other harmful consequences. Drugs are considered inappropriate chemical restraints when they are

- Given without specific indications
- Prescribed in excessive dosages, which affect an older adult's ability to function properly
- Used as sole treatment without investigating alternative, non-pharmacological, or behavioral interventions
- Administered for purposes of discipline or convenience of the staff

Many cases of inappropriate psychoactive drug use result either from the mistaken belief that these medications represent the only way of managing behaviors or from the fact that they are used as a substitute for adequate treatment.

Whether psychoactive medications are used as therapeutic agents or as restraints may be difficult to determine. For example, a psychoactive drug may be prescribed to treat agitated behavior, and its use results in an increased fall risk. The psychoactive drug is considered a therapeutic agent if it controls the individual's behavior and eliminates the risk of falls without restricting his or her ability to function; it is deemed a restraint if the person's activities (e.g., getting out of bed, going to the bathroom, engaging in social activities) are inhibited. Other medications used by older adults may be considered to be chemical restraints. For instance, some medications such as nonsteroidal anti-inflammatory drugs (analgesics), antihypertensives, and cardiotonics (cardiac drugs) prescribed for physical ailments can produce side effects such as disorientation, confusion, dizziness, and orthostatic hypotension or low blood pressure. In addition, polypharmacy (i.e., taking four or more medications) is common among older people. Any adverse interactions between drugs such as increased sedation or loss of coordination can result in cognitive and mobility impairments.

Aside from chemical restraints, the side effects of psychoactive drugs are particularly taxing on the physiological systems of older people. These side effects may include increased drowsiness, delirium or disordered thinking, low blood pressure, and Parkinsonian symptoms such as muscle rigidity in the limbs and gait disturbances. Such conditions may not only lead to further disruptive behavior but also increase the risk of falls and hip fractures. Also, psychoactive drugs may produce paradoxical agitation (i.e., rather than calming down a person, the drugs can sometimes increase agitation) in some older individuals, which clouds the issue of whether to increase or decrease drug dosages. Any increase of medication is likely to result in a vicious circle of higher doses and decreased functional ability.

Health care providers must take several steps before using psychoactive medications in patients and residents who present with cognitive disturbances, behavior disturbances, or both; they must identify the disturbance or specific symptom, and, if possible, discover the cause of the disturbance. Assessment of the underlying conditions responsible may eliminate the need for psychoactive medications. For example, confusion leading to disoriented behavior, agitation, or falling episodes may be due to an underlying infection or pharmacotoxicity. Thus, giving an antibiotic to clear the infection or stopping the medication is more appropriate than giving a psychoactive. Other common causes of disturbed behavior and changes in cognitive function in older people are the presence of pain, fecal impaction, metabolic abnormalities, and acute exasperation of chronic diseases. Also, simple events such as a wet bed, a room that is too hot or too cold, and hunger or thirst should not be overlooked as causes of behavior disturbances. Attempts should be made to reverse or eliminate the underlying cause through nonpharmacological approaches. In many instances, intervention with corrective behavioral and/or environmental strategies eliminates the need for psychoactive drugs. For instance, a succession of stressful events such as declining health, episodes of falling, admission to a hospital or a nursing facility, and the possibility of long-term institutional placement can bring about a complete breakdown of coping mechanisms, causing confusion. In such a situation, the provision of proper psychosocial counseling in dealing with the underlying stress may be beneficial in reversing the confusion. Likewise, allowing patients and residents to wander and providing a safe walking area may be all that is required to alleviate agitated behaviors.

During the period in which the underlying cause is being investigated, the patient or resident may continue to exhibit disturbed behaviors. To protect the individual from injuring him- or herself or others, it may be necessary to use a psychoactive drug in order to gain control over anxiety or aggression. In addition, if alternative approaches to eliminating the disturbed behavior are unsuccessful, psychoactive drugs may be required to improve the older individual's quality of life. Under such circumstances, obtaining a comprehensive drug history to guard against additive adverse effects and conducting laboratory studies to detect any hepatic or renal abnormalities that may influence the metabolism and excretion or elimination of the drug(s) must precede the use of psychoactive drugs. When a psychoactive is initiated, the prescriber should start with a low or small dose to test the person's responsiveness. Then the dosage should be increased slowly until the desired level of control is achieved without unwanted side effects. To ensure that psychoactive medications are used properly, staff should monitor patients and residents frequently for drug effectiveness and evidence of side effects. If drug therapy is unsuccessful or if the individual experiences adverse effects from the therapy, the medication should be discontinued and the plan of care revised. Also, staff must evaluate continually whether the person's disturbed behaviors have ceased or decreased in severity. In such an instance, staff should consider stopping the medication or reducing the dosage of the drug in order to avoid the risk of chemical restraint.

In summary, institutionally based health care providers play a major role in keeping patients and residents free of mechanical and chemical restraints. To meet this objective, providers should avoid the use of mechanical restraints to control falls and, instead, attempt restraint alternatives. Staff should not expose older adults who have never used psychoactive medications to these drugs unless they have a specific condition that calls for the medication. In addition, staff should reduce the dosage for individuals already using psychoactive drugs with the intent of stopping the drug, unless such a course is contraindicated clinically.

ENDNOTES

1. A mechanical restraint is defined as any mechanical device, material, or equipment attached or adjacent to the individual's body that the person cannot remove easily and is used to inhibit free, independent movement. These devices include vest and chest jackets or harnesses, waist belts and sheets, leg ties, full-length bed side rails, wheelchair safety bars, and geri-chairs with fixed tray tables.
2. Omnibus Budget Reconciliation Act (OBRA) of 1989, PL 101-239, 42 U.S.C. §§ 1396 *et seq.*
3. All such rationale supporting the use of mechanical restraints are based on myth, not reality.
4. Werner, P., Cohen-Mansfield, J., Braun, J., & Marx, M.S. (1989). Physical restraints and agitation in nursing home residents. *Journal of the American Geriatrics Society, 37*, 1122–1126.
5. Tinetti, M.E., Liu, W.L., & Ginter, S.F. (1992). Mechanical restraint use and fall-related injury among residents of skilled nursing facilities. *Annals of Internal Medicine, 116*, 369–374.

guidelines
and forms

part a

guidelines

best clinical practices in acute care hospitals and nursing facilities

PURPOSE

To provide a summary of best clinical practices to prevent patient falls in hospitals and nursing facilities, the most frequently occurring factors that increase fall risk, and the most commonly used interventions that reduce fall risk. Best clinical practices are simply ideas that work. Best practices in terms of fall prevention are strategies or interventions and practices that produce effective outcomes and decrease falls and injury. By knowing what causes falls and what strategies prevent falls, facilities can develop programs and protocols aimed at eliminating falls.

BEST PRACTICES IN ACUTE CARE HOSPITALS

The first part of this chapter deals with best clinical practices in acute care hospitals. Best practices of nursing facilities are discussed beginning on page 136.

Risk Factors

While many older patients are at some degree of risk of falling, certain factors have been consistently identified with high risk of falling. These include the intrinsic, extrinsic, and patient risk factors.

Intrinsic Risk Factors

- Age: Elderly patients older than age 75
- History of falling: Reported fall(s) during hospitalization; patients tend to repeat the circumstances of the first fall in subsequent falls
- Mental status: Impaired cognition—confusion, disorientation, poor memory, and inability to understand
- Medications: Psychotropic drugs such as sedatives and tranquilizers
- Dizziness or vertigo
- Lower extremity weakness
- Impaired mobility: Impaired transfers, gait/balance impairment
- Altered elimination: Urinary/bowel incontinence, urgency

Extrinsic Risk Factors

- Equipment issues: Broken wheelchair locks, bed wheels not locked
- Floor surfaces/treatments that promote slips
- Raised beds
- Full-length bed side rails
- Furnishings: Unstable chairs/over-the-bed tables

Patient Risk Factors

- Multiple risk factors (i.e., presence of more than one risk factor; risk increases as number of risk factors increases)
- Diagnoses:
    —Congestive heart failure (due to generalized weakness, nocturia)
    —Stroke (due to extremity weakness, aphasia/communication impairment)
    —Neoplasm (due to generalized weakness, side effects of anti-cancer drugs)

Most Frequent Causes/Sites of Patient Falls

- Transfers on and off beds (account for up to 50% of falls)
- Elimination (i.e., trips to bathroom)
- Types of units (unit-specific risk factors):
    —Psychiatry (depression, dementia, anxiety, antidepressants, orthostatic hypotension, wandering, aggressive behavior)
    —Rehabilitation units (incontinence, polypharmacy, stroke)
- Disability requiring assistance with activities of daily living [ADLs], and impaired wheelchair transfers

Assessment of Risk

Fall risk assessment tools should be employed to identify risk factors. By identifying specific fall risk factors, appropriate interventions aimed at minimizing risk can be identified and implemented. Risk assessments should be completed at the time of admission (within 24 hours) and, thereafter, whenever patients experience a change of status (i.e., acute illness, change in function, a move to another hospital unit).

Facilities can either use available risk assessment tools or develop their own risk assessments and incorporate them into the admission form for initial assessment and into the daily nursing assessment form for continual risk evaluation. Although established risk assessment tools are beneficial in identifying risk, tailoring risk assessments is helpful in meeting the unique needs of patient populations in specialty units (e.g., intensive care units, rehabilitation, telemetry, psychiatry).

Fall Preventive Interventions[1]

Staff Related

- Providing education (increasing awareness of patient fall risk during hospitalization and strategies to reduce risk)
- Communicating "at-risk" status (identifying fall risk status in patient's medical/nursing charts)

Patient Related

- Providing education (increasing patient/family awareness of fall risk during hospitalization and strategies to reduce risk)
- Attempting medication reduction (regularly reviewing patient medications/eliminating high-risk drugs as appropriate)
- Moving confused patients near nurses' station (close observation)
- Using sitters to sit with confused patients
- Using bed alarms (to alert staff when at-risk patients are attempting unsafe mobility tasks)
- Using identification bracelets (to identify high-risk patients)
- Using nonskid footwear
- Meeting elimination needs (placing patients near toilets, using bedside commodes, routine toileting schedules)

- Providing ambulation programs (e.g., walking high-risk patients in hallway once per shift)

Environment Related

- Keeping bed in low position, bed wheels locked
- Using half side rails as enablers (side rails to prevent falls is not successful)
- Reducing pathway clutter around patient's bed/bedroom
- Maintaining stable furnishings (beds/chairs used to maintain balance; help with efficient transfers)
- Improving lighting (nightlights at bedside/toilet)
- Installing toilet grab rails (to support safe transfers)

BEST PRACTICES IN NURSING FACILITIES

While all nursing facility residents are at some degree of risk of falling, certain factors have been consistently identified with high-risk of falling.* These include the following:

Risk Factors

Intrinsic Risk Factors

- History of falling: Reported fall(s) previous to institutionalization and/or during institutionalization
- Mental status: Impaired cognition—confusion, disorientation, poor memory, and inability to understand; dementia
- Vision impairment: Glaucoma, cataracts, macular degeneration, and functional vision loss
- Medications: Use of antidepressants and sedatives; use of more than four medications (i.e., polypharmacy)
- Post-prandial hypotension
- Lower extremity weakness
- Impaired mobility (e.g., impaired transfers, gait/balance impairment)

---

*Because the population of residents is similar or the same as that represented in the hospital practices listed previously, some of these risk factors are the same or similar.

- Assistive devices (e.g., canes, walkers)
- Toileting needs (i.e., urinary/bowel incontinence, urgency)
- Use of restraints

Extrinsic Risk Factors

- Equipment issues (e.g., wheelchair wheels not locked, bed wheels not locked)
- Slippery or wet floors
- Raised beds
- Inadequate assistive devices (e.g., canes, walkers)
- Lack of toilet grab rails
- Malfunctioning nurse call systems
- Use of full-length side rails

Patient Risk Factors[2]

- Presence of multiple risk factors (e.g., residents of advanced age with accompanying multiple chronic diseases, polypharmacy, cognitive impairment, and/or unsteady gait/balance)
- Diagnoses:
  —Congestive heart failure (presumably causes generalized weakness, nocturia)
  —Stroke (may cause extremity weakness, aphasia/communication impairment)
  —Parkinson's disease (may cause associated gait/balance impairment)
  —Degenerative joint disease (may cause associated lower extremity weakness)

Most Frequent Causes/Sites of Patient Falls

- Transfers on and off beds (account for up to 50% of falls)
- Elimination; trips to bathroom
- Transfers on and off chairs/wheelchairs

Assessment of Risk

Fall risk assessment tools can be employed to identify risk factors. The Minimum Data Set (MDS) contains some—but not all—of the information relevant to assessing fall risk. By identifying specific fall-risk factors (both intrinsic and extrinsic), appropriate interventions aimed at minimizing risk can be identified and implemented. Facilities either use available risk assessment tools or develop their own risk assessments and incorporate them into the admission form for initial assessment, and into the daily nursing assessment form for continual risk evaluation.

The Resident Assessment Protocols (RAPs) provide some information about fall risk (e.g., previous falls, medications/recent medication changes, assistive devices, environmental factors, neuromuscular/functional factors, orthopedic factors, sensory factors, and cognitive/behavioral factors). This information can be used to supplement risk factors identified on the fall risk assessment.

A fall risk assessment for all residents should be completed upon admission (within 24 hours) to the nursing facility, on a regular basis (i.e., to coincide with the MDS and/or whenever residents experience a change in condition), and post-fall.

Every time a resident falls, an assessment of the details or circumstances of the fall, causes of the fall, and contributing intrinsic and extrinsic factors should occur. The information obtained can be used to develop interventions to prevent further falls.

Recognize that using assessments to predict fall risk is not an exact science (i.e., some low-risk residents will fall and some high-risk residents may not fall). An effective fall risk assessment, however, should anticipate risk accurately more often than not.

Fall Preventive Interventions[3]

Staff Related

- Providing education (increasing awareness of patient fall risk during hospitalization and strategies to reduce risk)
- Communicating "at-risk" status (identifying fall risk status in patient's medical/nursing charts; reporting risk status at time of shift changes).
- Examining staffing patterns and maintaining adequate staff to assist high-risk residents
- Anticipating need of high-risk residents
- Monitoring high-risk residents (frequently observe fall-risk residents during the first week of institutional stay)

- Monitoring fall-risk residents during acute illnesses (represents high-risk time for falling)
- Monitoring residents during post-fall period (risk of further falls is increased)
- Developing an interdisciplinary falls consultation team to address high-risk residents with multiple falls
- Developing fall incident reports (ones that incorporate circumstances of falls/interventions)
- Developing an "Eyes/Ears" program aimed at early detection of fall risk (see Eyes and Ears Program, page 161)

Resident Related

- Attempting medication reduction (regularly reviewing patient's medications, eliminating high-risk drugs as appropriate)
- Moving confused patients near nurses' station (close observation)
- Using sitters to sit with confused patients
- Using bed alarms (to alert staff when at-risk patients are attempting unsafe mobility tasks)
- Using identifiers such as bracelets, stickers, or special socks (to identify high-risk patients)
- Having patients/residents use nonskid footwear
- Meeting elimination needs (placing patients near toilets, using bedside commodes, routine toileting schedules)
- Providing assistive devices (canes, walkers), as appropriate
- Providing supervised ambulation programs (walking high-risk patients in hallway once per shift)
- Providing exercise programs (chair-based exercises, stretching/ flexibility programs, and targeted strengthening exercises)
- Using hip protectors/pads (to reduce risk for hip fractures)
- Using gait belts to assist residents with unsteady transfers, ambulation, and balance
- Avoiding physical and chemical restraints (e.g, including use of side rails solely to prevent falls)

Environment Related

- Keeping beds in low position or using low platform beds
- Placing mats on floor along the bedside to reduce risk for injurious falls
- Keeping bed wheels locked or replacing wheels with immobilizer legs

- Using half side rails as enablers to support bed mobility
- Reducing pathway clutter around patient's bed/bedroom
- Maintaining stable furnishings (beds/chairs used to maintain balance; help with efficient transfers)
- Improving lighting (nightlights at bedside/toilet) and access to light switches
- Installing toilet grab rails (to support safe transfers)
- Installing carpeting on floor (avoids slipping on linoleum flooring)
- Maintaining wheelchair safety (removing/fixing broken wheelchairs)
- Providing frequent rest areas along hallways and other areas where residents ambulate
- Evaluating all assistive devices to ensure that they are the appropriate types

ENDNOTES

1. Despite considerable research addressing falls in acute care hospitals, it remains somewhat unclear as to what interventions are most effective in preventing falls. Based on fall risk assessments, designing targeted, multiple interventions is the most effective way to reduce risk, especially for high-risk patients.
2. High-risk factors may differ somewhat from institution to institution.
3. Care planning by an interdisciplinary team soon after admission to design targeted, multiple interventions is the most effective way to reduce fall risk in high-risk patients.

fall risk assessment

PURPOSE

- To outline the approach of managing patients/residents who are at risk for falls
- To provide staff with guidance for decisions regarding fall avoidance

STEPS

Step 1: Problem Definition

Decide whether the patient/resident is at fall risk. Common problems placing individuals at fall risk include the following:

- History of recent fall(s)
- Polypharmacy
- Cognitive impairment
- Bladder or bowel dysfunction
- Sensory changes (vision and hearing)
- Unsteady gait/balance
- Mobility impairment

Step 2: Assessment/Problem Analysis

Complete a fall risk assessment to identify what factors place patients/residents at fall risk. Formal risk assessments should be completed at the time of admission (within 24 hours) and thereafter whenever patients/residents experience a significant change in condition (i.e., onset of acute illness, worsening of chronic diseases, medication changes). Fall risk assessment tools help to identify whether patients/residents are at risk for falling. In order to ensure staff compliance with risk evaluation, and the likelihood of the tool being effective in terms of falls reduction, fall risk assessment tools should

- Be quick to complete and simple to use
- Include the most common factors related to falls, including a functional and environmental assessment
- Be able to identify patients/residents "at risk" or with a "high risk" of falling
- Use prompts to initiate referrals aimed at further in-depth interdisciplinary assessments, and contain immediate actions or interventions aimed at fall avoidance

In addition to formal risk assessments, staff should assess patients/residents

- Each day for ability to transfer/ambulate
- Each shift for change of condition/environmental hazards
- Any time that a fall risk is observed (such as acute illness and/or changes in mental status)

In those patients/residents with falls

- Assess the patient/resident for injury (e.g., pain, abrasions, bruises, fractures)
- Identify circumstances surrounding the fall. Often, identifying and correcting the cause of a fall can reduce the likelihood of subsequent falls
- Communicate high-risk fall status to all members of the patient's/resident's interdisciplinary team

Step 3: Problem Management

Use the information gathered to decide and plan how best to manage the patient's/resident's problems (i.e., what causes or risk factors are correctable). As patients/residents may have several fall risk factors, designing a care plan aimed at preventing falls is most effective when achieved through an interdisciplinary approach.

Step 4: Monitoring

Regularly evaluate the patient's/resident's progress (i.e., effectiveness of interventions and/or the need to redesign interventions).

SAMPLE TOOL

No single fall risk assessment tool meets the needs of every facility. Health professionals will either have to choose from the wide variety of risk assessment tools already available or create their own tools. Although the effectiveness of fall risk assessment tools is somewhat controversial (i.e., some tools identify a high percentage of patients/residents at risk), the real value of a risk assessment tool is that it raises staff awareness of patients/residents who are at risk of falling, and staff awareness of risk is an important first step in preventing falls. Table II-2 on page 144 includes an example of the most relevant risk factors and immediate safety interventions that should be included in a fall risk assessment tool. The goal of the form is not to determine the cause(s) of risk or impairments, which should occur during routine multidisciplinary assessment and plan of care, but to provide at-risk patients/residents with *immediate* safety. Section Two, Part B includes a Fall Risk Checklist that is also helpful.

Further information/copies of fall and fall risk guidelines can be obtained from

- American Medical Directors Association (800-876-2632; www. amda.com)
- University of Iowa Nursing Interventions Research Center, Department of Nursing-RDDC, 4118 Westlawn, Iowa City, IA 52242–1100

Table II-2. Risk factors and recommended interventions

Risk factors	Specific types of risks	Recommended interventions
Medications	Medication changes within 24 hours Anticholinergics Antipsychotics Diuretics Sedatives	Physician evaluation (drug review) Pharmacist evaluation (drug/drug and drug/food interactions) Monitor postural blood pressure (sitting/standing)
Cognitive impairments	Disorientation/ delirium Dementia Depression Anxiety Impaired communication Impaired judgment	Physician evaluation Frequent observation checks Assess need to utilize sitters Assess need for bed alarms Consider moving confused patient/resident near nurses' station
History of recent fall(s)	Injurious fall(s) Fear of falling	Physician evaluation Identify/communicate "at-risk" for falls Frequent observation checks
Bladder dysfunction	Incontinence Nocturia Frequency	Physician evaluation Evaluate toileting needs/routines Consider placing patients/residents with urgency near toilets Assess need for bedside commode Consider nightlights at bedside/toilet
Sensory changes	Impaired vision Impaired hearing	Physician evaluation Provide easy access to glasses/ hearing aids Observe mobility in patients/residents environment; note any difficulties encountered and modify as needed

Table II-2. *(continued)*

Risk factors	Specific types of risks	Recommended interventions
Postural hypotension/ dizziness	Cardiovascular diseases/ medication	Physician evaluation Orthostatic vital sign checks Assess need for assistance with transfers
Unsteady gait/balance	Stroke Parkinson's disease Musculoskeletal conditions Neuromuscular conditions Foot problems	Physician evaluation Physical therapy evaluation Assistive devices (cane, walker) Assist with ambulation as needed Evaluate footwear safety (consider nonslip socks/footwear)
Mobility impairment	Transfer impairment Ambulation impairment Ambulation device (cane, walker)	Physician evaluation Physical therapy evaluation Place bed in low position Consider using side rails as enablers Assist with ambulation/transfers as needed Consider use of chair/bed alarms Keep call bell within reach Evaluate safety of ambulation devices Environmental evaluation (e.g., bedroom and furnishings, bathroom, surrounding hazardous conditions), modify as needed

fall prevention and restraint avoidance programs

PURPOSE

A commitment to patient and resident safety requires a clearly defined, coordinated, and ongoing Fall Prevention and Restraint Avoidance (FPRA) program. The goals of any FPRA program are

- To prevent and/or reduce the risk of falls and fall-related injury
- To promote patient/resident mobility and autonomy
- To avoid the use of restraints to maintain safety

STRUCTURE

Structure and *process* represent the basic building blocks of a successful FPRA program, whether it is housed in an acute care hospital or a nursing facility. Structure refers to the "who"—the individuals needed to accomplish a program, and the "what"—the resources needed to achieve success or positive outcomes. Process refers to the "how"—the care-planning steps needed to achieve positive outcomes. Putting the two together, structure plus process equals *outcomes*. Outcomes refer to the set of goals one hopes to accomplish by having a fall prevention program in place, including reduced falls and injurious falls, reduced use of physical restraints, and enhanced mobility. The basic components for a comprehensive fall prevention and restraint reduction program follow.

Knowledge and Expertise of Health Professionals

- Educate all staff on why it is important to assess for fall risk and restraint-use risk (e.g., on the potentially harmful effects of restraints), and provide clear guidance on how and when to assess risk (e.g., once per shift, daily, only when there is a change in condition and/or medications).
- Educate all staff on the relationship between fall risk and risk for restraint use and the contributory factors for both. Staff awareness of this relationship is crucial in order to produce effective strategies.
- Educate all staff on available facility strategies for reducing/ preventing falls and restraint use. Any time new devices or equipment, such as bed alarms and/or least-restraining appliances are introduced into the facility, staff should receive education and training on their benefits and how to use them properly and safely.
- Educate all staff on the institutional definition of what counts as a fall; for instance, only witnessed falls or "near falls" such as observed episodes of an individual experiencing imbalance or of being assisted down to the floor or into a chair or bed following imbalance, and unwitnessed events such as "found down on the floor." In general, an episode where the patient or resident experienced imbalance and would have fallen were it not for staff intervention or the support of walls and furnishings should be counted. Similar to actual falls, episodes of imbalance and/or "found down" can represent the first sign or symptom of an underlying intrinsic and/or extrinsic problem requiring evaluation. By correcting the underlying cause of the problem, an actual fall may be prevented from occurring. The importance of reporting both falls and near falls is to identify and communicate problems and potential problems in order to implement interventions.
- Educate all staff on why falls occur and how to evaluate patients/ residents with falls (e.g., using a process of root cause analysis that attempts to identify the intrinsic, extrinsic, and organizational or process factors causative of falls).
- Educate all staff on safety policies and procedures related to fall prevention and restraint avoidance. This education should begin

at the time of a staff member's orientation and should be ongoing. It is important that aides, orderlies, and those individuals providing custodial services (e.g., housekeeping, maintenance) receive education as well because they can notice patients/residents early on who may be at fall risk; for example, they may be the first to observe the onset of an individual's confusion or unsteady balance. In addition, the roles and responsibilities of each staff member need to be spelled out in terms of what they can do to prevent falls.

Number and Type of Health Professionals

Examine the number and type of health professionals needed. The precise number of staff needed is highly dependent on the number of patients/residents at fall risk and number of staff available to provide care (i.e., patient/resident mix). The type of staff includes all multidisciplinary staff needed to accomplish the fall prevention and restraint-avoidance program.

Physical Environment and Resources

- Examine the elements of the physical environment that might be placing older individuals at risk. The physical environment includes the structure of units (e.g., beds; furniture placement; types/conditions of walking surfaces; lighting/glare; safety or grab bars in hallways, bathrooms, and common areas). Environmental hazards can contribute to falls, especially in high-risk patients/residents, and interventions or modification of identified hazards can reduce risk of falling.
- Determine resources needed. Resources include availability of equipment and devices to reduce falls and restraint use (e.g., bed alarms, ambulation devices and wheelchairs, bedside commodes, wedge pillows/cushions and other positioning cushions, nonslip socks, bed transfer bars, non-restraint alternative devices). A lack of resources can contribute to falls and restraint use, and conversely, maintaining adequate resources can assist with safe mobility and can reduce the risk of falls and restraint use.

Leadership Support

Organizational leadership support (e.g., from department heads, senior management, and administration) for the FPRA program is crucial in order to move any risk reduction or avoidance practices forward. The benefits of strong leadership include

- Providing adequate resources such as staff and equipment so that interventions can be implemented
- Providing support for staff education
- Helping to break down barriers between departments so that staff work together in a multidisciplinary manner
- Ensuring dissemination of the FPRA program throughout the facility, and supporting a systemic approach to designing, implementing, analyzing, and improving efforts to prevent falls and reduce restraints
- Fostering a "culture of safety" throughout the facility (i.e., communicating the importance of fall prevention and restraint avoidance within the facility). A culture of safety includes making it safer or non-punitive for staff to report falls.

Not all falls are reflections of poor or substandard care because patients and residents who fall may show no evidence of risk for falling (e.g., when a fall is due to an unanticipated acute illness). In turn, promoting a culture of safety will result in positive attitudes and "buy-in" by staff toward the FPRA program.

Protocols and Guidelines

Facilities should have protocols and guidelines governing the FPRA program (i.e., systematically developed statements to assist staff and patient/resident decisions about the care-planning process with respect to fall prevention and restraint reduction activities). All staff need to be regularly oriented and educated to the protocols and guidelines. The most effective protocols and guidelines

- Are straightforward, explaining who does what and when they should do it, and easy for staff to follow
- Are readily available for staff

- Describe the most common risk factors/interventions related to falls and restraint use
- Are updated periodically

Falls/Restraint Prevention Committee

Setting up a falls/restraint prevention committee is beneficial. The purpose of this committee, comprised of multidisciplinary representatives from medicine, nursing, rehabilitation, pharmacy, and social services, is to investigate falls (i.e., research the circumstances of patients and residents with injurious falls, multiple falls, or those experiencing excessive restraint use) and make recommendations for safety. In addition, it is recommended that maintenance, custodial, or housekeeping personnel also be involved in the process because facilities' layout and maintenance (e.g., lighting levels, floor conditions, broken equipment) contribute to falls.

Within the committee, identify a falls coordinator and a team leader. The falls coordinator should be an individual with knowledge and experience in falls and restraints; one who is able to provide the committee with guidance and reference resources as needed. The team leader should be an individual who is well respected in the facility (such as the director of nursing or medical director); one who can help the committee move forward within the facility. The committee may have several functions:

- Review and analyze institutional falls/restraints (e.g., incidence of fall/injurious fall frequency and restraint use; fall/injurious fall and restraint circumstances). This information will help determine causes of falls and restraint use as well as actions that can be taken to reduce falls and restraints.
- Review and revise (as needed) the current facility fall risk/restraint reduction process (i.e., identify risk and available interventions and care planning), and fall reporting mechanisms including the effectiveness of incident reports.
- Educate staff about falls and restraints. Organize a staff orientation program on fall prevention and restraint reduction, to include precautions to take and methods for preventing falls and avoiding restraints, and education on fall- and restraint-related policies, procedures, and protocols.

- Review and disseminate current government regulations related to falls and restraints, and revise policies and procedures accordingly to ensure facility compliance with regulatory mandates.

STEPS

Step 1: Risk Identification

The most important action that hospitals and nursing facilities can take is to identify an individual's risk for falls at the time he or she is admitted. To say that all older patients and residents are at risk for falls is basically true but somewhat meaningless because some patients and residents are more at risk than others. Therefore, each patient and resident should receive a falls risk assessment that uncovers factors and combinations of factors that place him or her at fall risk.

Risk assessments should address both intrinsic factors (i.e., related to the individual) and extrinsic factors (i.e., related to the environment). When health care professionals identify and correct risk factors, the majority of falls can be prevented. Hospitals and nursing facilities may choose different methods to identify fall-risk individuals. (See pages 133–134 and 136–137 for a list of risk factors.)

Facilities should have a method for all staff to recognize patients and residents at high risk for falls. Visual reminders of patients/residents who are "at risk," such as colored identification bands, colored nonslip socks, and/or bedroom door and bed stickers indicating "at risk" are the most commonly used ways of identifying patients/residents at fall risk. Wrist identification bands and nonslip socks are the most effective because they are a portable method of identification; wherever "at-risk" patient/residents are on the unit, staff will recognize them.

Facility staff should investigate all falls and complete a written report for each. Incident or occurrence reports should include circumstances of the fall, responsible causes or contributing factors, and presence of any injury. A reassessment of fall risk should be done post-fall, since the patient/resident may have new risk factors.

Step 2: Develop a Care Plan

After completing the risk assessment, staff should develop a care plan for patients/residents with specific, individualized interventions matched to identified fall risk factors. The care plan should identify various risk factors that increase the likelihood of falls and restraint use, interdisciplinary interventions aimed at reducing fall and restraint-use risk, intervention goals, responsible disciplines for completing the interventions, and a time frame for evaluating the effectiveness of interventions. If falls continue to occur, consider other possible reasons for fall risk besides those already identified. For those patients and residents who fall repeatedly and/or require restraints (i.e., where the cause cannot be modified or controlled), identify ways to reduce the risk of injurious falls and restraint complications.

Step 3: Follow-Up

Evaluate and re-evaluate outcomes or the effectiveness of interventions included in the care plan on a continual basis, and revise the patient's/resident's plan of care as needed. Steps of a good follow-up plan include the following:

- Complete a fall and restraint risk assessment whenever a patient/ resident experiences a change of condition and/or states problems with imbalance, mobility, and so forth.
- Observe and communicate "at-risk" status (includes keeping an eye on patients/residents, particularly those individuals at risk, and communicating with physicians and ancillary providers regarding the current risk status of patients/residents).
- Document and evaluate all falls when they occur to see what other interventions can be put into place to prevent falls.

Step 4: Evaluation

Monitor and measure fall rates and restraint use rates over time. Trending falls and restraint use is of benefit from two perspectives: evaluating the effectiveness of FPRA programs, and assessing patient/ resident outcomes (i.e., whether fall and restraint rates have decreased).

Methods for calculating fall rates and restraint use rates are listed in Measuring Fall Rates and Restraint Use Rates (pp. 157–160). Audit the process of care. This step is crucial, especially if no improvements in falls and/or restraint use occur. Information obtained can help to determine areas for improvement. Documentation should reflect steps in the care-planning process (e.g., consistently using fall-risk tools, identifying risk factors and appropriate interventions in the patient's/resident's care plan), the benefits of interventions, and the patient's or resident's response.

Provide staff with regular feedback on the audit results, especially if positive. Staff are more likely to be compliant with the care-planning process if they know that their efforts are improving care.

Critical steps in determining the effectiveness of a facility's care planning process include a review of the facility's policies and procedures that govern the care-planning process. Evaluating the process of care in conjunction with analysis of falls and restraint data assists facilities in creating a cycle of continuous improvement (i.e., changes or modifications continue to be made in the FPRA program in response to the audit's results).

BARRIERS TO A SUCCESSFUL FALL PREVENTION AND RESTRAINT AVOIDANCE PROGRAM

Certain situational factors or hidden disaster risks always exist to a certain extent in any facility that can hinder the care-planning process or implementation of strategies intended to prevent falls. Any breakdown in structure and process has the potential to make the difference between an organized versus an unorganized process, and whether good versus poor outcomes occur. As well, any failure in process can expose facilities to liability risk. By identifying structure and process problems, facilities can greatly improve the care-planning process and increase the likelihood of reducing the risk of falls and avoiding restraints. Some of the most important structural and process barriers interfering with successful outcomes include

- Poorly trained staff (i.e., those with a lack of knowledge about risk assessment, procedures, and/or preventive interventions)
- Inadequate or inaccurate risk assessments

- Sub-optimal or lack of communication among staff related to patient/resident risk
- Lack of chart documentation related to patient/resident risk
- Delayed multidisciplinary referrals (i.e., further evaluation by necessary professional or trained staff of patient/resident risk and/or identification of underlying problems)
- Staff shortages
- Inadequate staff/patient and resident ratios (i.e., insufficient staff to properly care for the number of patients/residents requiring care)
- Constant staff turnover
- Delayed or insufficient medical and nursing care
- Reduced use of restraints without available nonrestraint alternatives
- Malfunction of equipment (e.g., nurse call system, bed alarm systems, bed wheel locking systems, wheelchairs)
- Lack of established policies and procedures regarding falls and restraint prevention
- Staff noncompliance with protocols/procedures
- Inadequate resources (e.g., bed alarm devices, assistive devices, non-restraint alternatives)

restraint/non-restraint utilization assessment

PURPOSE

- To outline the approach to managing patients/residents who are at risk for physical restraint use
- To provide staff with guidance for decisions regarding the use of physical restraints and non-restraint use

STEPS

Step 1: Problem Definition

Decide whether there is a problem indicating need for physical restraint use. Common reasons for physical restraint use include

- Falls/fall risk
- Unsafe wandering
- Agitated behavior
- Interference with medical treatment (i.e., use of tubes, intravenous lines, catheters, and so forth)

Step 2: Assessment/Problem Analysis

- Identify the root cause of the problem or what is causing the patient's/resident's behavior.
- Talk to the patient/resident in order to determine circumstances surrounding the behavior.

- Review the patient's/resident's health problems and medications.
- Identify factors that place the patient/resident at risk for restraint use.

Step 3: Problem Management

- Decide how to best manage the patient's/resident's condition (i.e., which causes are correctable or modifiable and which conditions require consideration of restraints or non-restraint alternatives).

Step 4: Monitoring

- Evaluate the patient's/resident's progress in relation to the problem and effectiveness of interventions.

SAMPLE TOOL

A blank restraint assessment tool that can be used to compile the most relevant information is included in Part B of Section Two. Further information/copies of physical restraint guidelines can be obtained from

- American Medical Directors Association (800-876-2632; www. amda.com)
- University of Iowa Nursing Interventions Research Center, Department of Nursing-RDDC, 4118 Westlawn, Iowa City, IA 52242-1100

measuring fall rates
and restraint use rates

PURPOSE

Measuring fall rates and restraint use rates in a standardized manner helps organizations to

- Monitor internal performance over time and trends in order to identify opportunities for improvement
- Compare rates with external organizations (e.g., organizations with "similar" populations) in order to provide target goals

Fall rates and restraint use rates are usually expressed as percentages and calculated by month and quarter, with comparisons throughout the year to show trends and relationships to fall-preventive and restraint-reduction activities.

Rate of Falls

The rate of falls is calculated by dividing the number of falls by the number of patient/resident days[1] and multiplying the resulting quotient by 100.

Number of Falls ÷ Number of Patient/Resident Days × 100 = Rate of Falls

Rate of Residents with Repeated Falls

The rate of patients/residents with repeated falls is calculated by dividing the number of patients/residents with more than one fall by the number of patients/residents experiencing one or more falls during the reported period and multiplying the quotient by 100.

Number of Patients/Residents with More Than One Fall ÷ Number of Patients/Residents Experiencing One or More Falls × 100 = Rate of Patients/Residents with Repeated Falls

Rate of Injurious Falls

The rate of injurious falls is calculated by dividing the number of injurious falls by the number of falls and multiplying the resulting quotient by 100.

Number of Injurious Falls ÷ Number of Falls × 100 = Rate of Injurious Falls

OTHER WAYS TO RATE FALLS

Several other ways to further stratify fall rates to assist organizations in determining risk factors and identifying opportunities for improvement are used:

- By unit type (e.g., rehabilitation, geropsychiatry, ICUs)
- By cause of falls (e.g., medical/functional conditions, medication types, environmental hazards, time of day, length of stay, location).

Physical Restraint-Use Rates

The rate of physical restraint events (defined as the period between restraint initiation time and release time) is calculated by dividing the number of physical restraint events by the number of patient/resident days[1] and multiplying the resulting quotient by 100.

Number of Physical Restraint Events ÷ Number of Patient/Resident Days × 100 = Rate of Physical Restraint-Use Events

Rate of Patients/Residents with Restraints

The rate of patients/residents with physical restraints is calculated by dividing the number of patients/residents with one or more physical restraint events by the number of patients/residents and multiplying the resulting quotient by 100.

Number of Patients/Residents with One or More Physical Restraints ÷ Number of Patients/Residents × 100 = Rate of Patients/Residents with Restraints

Rate of Repeated Restraint Use

The repeated restraint-use rate is calculated by dividing the number of patients/residents with more than one physical restraint event by the number of patients/residents with one or more physical restraint events and multiplying the resulting quotient by 100.

Number of Patients/Residents with More than One Physical Restraint Event ÷ Number of Patient/Residents with One or More Physical Restraint Events = Repeated Restraint-Use Rate

Rate of Duration of Physical Restraint Events

The rates for physical restraint events by specified duration[2] are calculated by dividing the number of physical restraint events for a specified duration by the total number of physical restraint events and multiplying the resulting quotient by 100.

Number of Physical Restraint Events by Specified Duration ÷ Number of Physical Restraint Events × 100 = Rate of Physical Restraint Events by Duration

Rate of Physical Restraint Events by Reason

The rates for physical restraint events by reason are calculated by dividing the number of physical restraint events by specified reason (e.g., to prevent falls, agitation) by the total number of physical restraint events and multiplying the resulting quotient by 100.

Number of Physical Restraint Events by Specified Reason ÷ Number of Physical Restraint Events × 100 = Rate of Physical Restraint Events by Reason

ENDNOTES

1. The "number of patient/resident days" is calculated by adding the number of patient/resident days, or census, for each calendar day of the month.
2. Restraint duration is the cumulative time from restraint initiation to restraint removal for each restraint event.

eyes and ears program

PURPOSE

To train staff to detect clinical change of not-yet-visible problems/illness and risk before falls occur; to prevent falls by heightening staff's awareness of patients/residents at high risk for falls. The more eyes available to watch older adults at high risk (e.g., observing warning signs such as unsteady balance or a change in condition such as agitation, confusion, weakness or tiredness, needing help with their daily activities) and the more ears available to hear the messages of high-risk older adults that indicate fall risk (e.g., listening to an individual talk about his or her symptoms, such as feeling dizzy or unwell, or problems with balance and/or functional activities), the better it is. Changes noted in an individual's behavior and functional activities can often serve as an early alerting mechanism to the clinical staff (e.g., to look for an underlying cause, disease/drug reaction) and help to prevent falls.

Who Should Watch

All facility employees who are in regular contact with patients/residents and/or their environments. This group should include nursing aides/assistants, housekeeping, dietary, laundry, clerical, maintenance, and administrative staff in addition to medical, nursing, rehabilitation, pharmacy, and social services staff who are already involved in daily care responsibilities. As well, available family members can be involved in the program.

Who Should Be Watched

Patients/residents most likely to benefit from an eyes and ears monitoring program include

- Frequent fallers (e.g., those with two or more falls)
- Frequent wanderers
- Patients/residents with dementia and gait/balance impairments

It is important to limit the number of patients to be monitored as part of the Eyes and Ears program because identifying too many patients/residents to monitor may desensitize staff from paying attention to those most at risk for falling.

STEPS

Step 1: Educate All Employees

Educate all employees about the program. Arrange a half-hour inservice presentation on the importance of fall prevention within the facility (i.e., for both the facility in terms of legal liability and patients/residents with regard to harmful consequences), the necessity for identifying patients/residents at fall risk, an explanation of the eyes and ears program, and what role or responsibilities employees have in the program. It's important to educate employees by sharpening their observational and listening skills while recognizing employee limitations. For example, maintenance employees can be taught to conduct weekly rounds to observe for environmental factors, such as lighting levels, floor conditions, broken or defective wheelchairs, bed brakes, and so forth.

Step 2: Formalize a Reporting System

Employees participating in the program need to have an established person with whom they can share their patient/resident and environmental observations (e.g., the head nurse).

Step 3: Determine the Patients/Residents Who Will Be Included

Identify patients and residents who should be included in the program and document their program participation in their chart.

Step 4: Visibly Identify "At-Risk" Program Participants

Identify at-risk program participants by a colorful identification wristband or sticker (e.g., a falling star or leaf). This enables employees to quickly identify patients and residents who are part of the program and at high risk for falling. A colorful identification wristband or sticker is a signal to observe the patient/resident closely and to intervene if the patient/resident displays any unsafe behaviors (getting up from bed without assistance) and/or voices any problems. This also helps alert staff who may not be familiar with patients/residents (such as agency nurses and other staff) to the individual's risk status. Affix the sticker

- By the patient's/resident's room
- Above the bed
- To his or her ambulation device (e.g., cane, walker, wheelchair)

Step 5: Identify Times of High Risk for Falls

Identify times when patients/residents may be most at risk for falls in order to anticipate their needs, such as before or right after meals; while going to the bathroom, getting out of or back into bed, or during toileting; late afternoon (because of shift changes, sundowning, or late afternoon confusion); or downtime between activities (because of boredom, patients/residents may become restless and try to get up from chairs/beds and fall). This alerts all employees in contact with the patients/residents that special care and supervision are required.

Step 6: Evaluation

Monitor outcomes of the Eyes and Ears program. This will help determine if the program and actions taken to reduce fall risk are effective.

ambulation device measurement

Cane Measurements

The measurement of cane height is the same regardless of cane type. Ask the person wearing everyday shoes to stand erect, with arms hanging loosely by his or her sides. The cane (or center of a multistem cane) is placed approximately 6 inches to the front and side of the person's shoe.

Two landmarks are used to determine proper height: the greater trochanter and the angle of the elbow. The top of the cane should come to approximately the level of the greater trochanter and the elbow should be flexed at 20°–30°. The degree of elbow flexion is the most important indicator of correct height because it allows the arm to shorten or lengthen during different phases of gait. This degree of flexion prevents the person from leaning forward or into the cane (if too short) or away, or leaning precariously backward (if too tall).

Walker Measurements

The measurement of walker height is similar to that of a cane. Place the walker 10–12 inches in front of the person's feet so that the walker partially surrounds the person. In this position, the handles should come to approximately the greater trochanter and the elbow is flexed at 20°–30°.

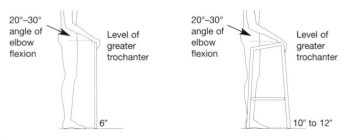

20°–30° angle of elbow flexion   Level of greater trochanter   6″

20°–30° angle of elbow flexion   Level of greater trochanter   10″ to 12″

ambulation device utilization

Cane Ambulation: Level Ground

For cane ambulation on level ground, the cane is held on the side of the body that is opposite to the affected limb. This position provides the greatest base of support and simulates normal gait. When the cane is held on the same side of the body as that of the affected limb, the person's center of gravity shifts from side to side. This position produces an abnormal, uncomfortable gait and leads to instability.

The cane and the involved extremity are advanced simultaneously (see figure on page 166). The cane is held relatively close to the body and should not be placed ahead of the affected limb. Placing the cane too far to the side or forward will cause lateral bending, forward bending, or both, resulting in a loss of stability.

Walker Ambulation: Level Ground

Standard Walker Ambulation using the standard walker on level ground requires the person to have enough stability to balance on one or both feet while he or she picks up the walker and moves it forward. The "step to" and "step through" gaits are the ones used most often for stability and to protect arthritic joints. Weight is placed on the hands (i.e., hands push down on walker) and, at the same time, the other, unaffected foot is moved forward, either parallel to ("step to" gait) or past ("step through" gait) the opposite, affected foot. The person should not step too close to the front bar of the walker because this motion decreases the base of support and may cause the person to fall backward.

Step pattern using cane.

Sliding Walker   The use of the sliding walker is similar to that of the standard walker, except that the sliding walker is not picked up but slid along the floor. A "step to" or "step through" gait is employed.

Rolling Walker   Weight is shifted from all four walker legs to the forward (wheeled) legs. The walker is rolled forward until the hands are 10–12 inches ahead of the feet. A "step to" or "step through" gait is employed.

Cane Ambulation: Turning

Turning is accomplished by moving to the unaffected side using a gait similar to that used when walking on level ground surfaces. To start, feet are kept slightly apart in order to maintain balance. The cane and feet are moved in a small circle. The following sequence is used: First, the cane and the affected limb are moved, then the unaffected limb is moved. The unaffected limb is kept on the inside of the circle. The person should not pivot on the unaffected limb to maintain his or her balance. The process is repeated until the turn is complete (see the figure on page 167).

Walker Ambulation: Turning

Turning with a walker is similar to that of turning with a cane. A "step to" or "step through" gait is employed.

Step pattern while turning with cane.

Cane Transfers: Standing

In making a cane transfer to the standing position, the person slides forward to the edge of his or her seat. The standard cane is placed against the chair armrest; the quad cane or hemi-walker cane is positioned in front of and to the unaffected side of the body. The person places his or her feet in the stride position (i.e., unaffected leg behind affected leg) with both hands on the armrests, leans forward and comes to a standing position, and then grasps the cane.

Walker Transfers: Standing

In making a walker transfer to the standing position, the person moves forward to the edge of his or her seat. The walker is positioned directly in front of the chair. The person places his or her feet in the stride position (i.e., unaffected leg behind affected leg), grasps both armrests of the chair, leans forward and comes to a standing position by pushing down on the armrests, and then reaches for the walker.

Cane Transfers: Sitting

In making a cane transfer to the sitting position, the person approaches the chair, turns in a small circle toward the unaffected side of the body, and backs up until the chair edge is felt against the legs. The person reaches for the chair armrest with his or her free hand, releases the broad-based cane or leans the standard cane against the chair, grasps the opposite armrest, and sits down.

Walker Transfers: Sitting

In making a walker transfer to the sitting position, the person approaches the chair, turns in a small circle toward the unaffected side of the body, and backs up until the chair edge is felt against the legs.

The person reaches for one chair armrest at a time, releases his or her grasp on the walker, and sits down.

bed safety

PURPOSE

To help care providers learn strategies for preventing falls from beds. One of the most common locations of falls in hospitals and nursing facilities is from bed, and the act of transferring in or out of bed is one of the most common causes of falls. The key to preventing falls from bed is for caregivers and patients to adhere to an organized process, which consists of the following.

STEPS

Step 1: Assessment

Bed mobility is best assessed by observing the patient/resident transferring from his or her bed and observing whether the individual is able to accomplish the task in a safe manner (see the Performance-Oriented Environmental Mobility Screen [POEMS] in Part B). This takes only a few minutes to complete and provides more useful information than simply asking patients/residents about whether they are able to transfer safely from bed. Some patients/residents overstate their transfer ability because they may feel embarrassed about having difficulty getting up from bed. Other patients/residents may think that their transfers are safe, when in fact they are hazardous. Finally, patients/residents with dementia and other communication impairments will not be able to accurately describe their bed transfers.

In those patients/residents exhibiting poor bed mobility, it is important to assess for any underlying diseases and/or medications that may be interfering with safe transfers and to treat any problems found. Strategies include management of active chronic diseases and discontinuation of all offending medications.

Step 2: Intervention

• Exercise programs aimed at improving upper/lower extremity strength and joint range of motion as well as balance performance can increase transfer skills.

• Maximizing transfer tasks by choosing beds that meet functional needs can help promote safe transfers and reduce the likelihood of falling. Adaptive strategies to make beds safer for patients/residents include 1) proper bed height to allow for safe transfers, 2) firm mattress to support sitting balance, 3) application of non-slip adhesive strips on the floor along the length of the bed for stable footing during transfers, and 4) locking bed wheels or using immobilizer legs to prevent the bed from rolling away during transfers.

Step 3: Consideration of Bed Side Rails

Some patients/residents will continue to remain at fall risk despite these interventions and/or bed modifications. Occasionally, side rails may be used to support safe bed activities. (See Side Rail Utilization Assessment Guidelines, which list the potential benefits of side rails.) When considering the use of a bed side rail, it is important to first assess the patient/resident and identify what, if any, factors place the individual at risk for problems related to side rail use (see Side Rail Utilization Assessment Guidelines). The indiscriminate use of side rails can be hazardous, but side rails can be both appropriate and beneficial when evaluated and considered through a well-thought-out, individualized assessment and plan of care involving patients/residents in the decision process as appropriate. Second, determine the following:

• Does the patient/resident want side rails?
• What is the intent of side rails (i.e., what do you want to accomplish)?
• What is the effect on the patient's/resident's function (i.e., will side rails hinder or assist mobility)?

- Will side rails prevent or facilitate what the patient/resident wants to do?
- Do the benefits of side rails outweigh the risks of potential harm for this individual?

Types of Side Rails

- Full-length side rails are most useful for patients/residents who are immobile because they prevent the individuals from rolling out of bed. The use of side rail pads or protective coverings can help to prevent injuries in patients/residents at risk for thrashing about while in bed, such as those with dementia.
- Half side rails are beneficial as enablers to assist patients/residents with poor bed mobility/transfers.
- Bed alarm systems, which alert staff to individuals who are leaving their beds so that staff can check on them immediately, may be used in conjunction with both full- and half-length rails to help detect fall risk and avoid falls early on.

Alternatives to Side Rails If side rails pose a risk of harm for an individual, some alternatives to consider include

- Equipping the bed with a trapeze bar to increase bed mobility
- Keeping the bed in the lowest position with bed wheels locked
- Using low platform beds or beds that can be lowered close to the floor
- Placing mats on the floor next to the bed to prevent falls from bed from being injurious (Caution: Individuals with gait/balance impairments may be at risk of tripping over the mat. For these individuals, placing the mat on the floor after the person is in bed and taking up the mat before they get out of bed may be tried.)

Step 4: Monitoring

- Anticipate the reasons patients/residents get out of bed, such as to go to the bathroom. By meeting the patient's/resident's needs, the risk of falls can be averted.
- Re-evaluate mobility on a regular basis, especially following falls.
- Re-evaluate the risks and possible effects of side rails against the risks and potential beneficial effects of alternatives to side rails.

As the patients/residents either improve or worsen, the indications for side rails are subject to change.

* Inspect bed frames, side rails, and mattresses regularly for potential entrapment hazards. It's important to use compatible side rails and mattresses to prevent gaps in which patients/residents could be entrapped. Beds, mattresses, and side rails are designed to fit together, but commonly, pieces are purchased separately and replaced as equipment wears out. This can leave gaps large enough to trap an individual between the mattress and side rail, putting the individual at risk of injury or suffocation.

side rail utilization assessment

PURPOSE

To assist staff in determining the appropriate use of side rails. Side rails can be regarded as physical restraints if they restrict the movement of a patient/resident, or as "enablers" if they support the bed mobility of a patient/resident. When side rails are used or considered to enable mobility, assessment should include a review of the following factors regarding a patient/resident:

- Bed mobility (i.e., does the side rail assist the patient/resident to turn from side to side while in bed or is the patient/resident totally immobile and unable to shift without assistance?)
- Bed transfers (i.e., does the side rail help the patient/resident get up safely from bed with minimal risk of falling?)

STEPS

- Step 1: Gather baseline data.
- Step 2: Describe rationale for potential side rail use.
- Step 3: Determine side rail use recommendations. Describe when and why side rails are used (i.e., how long and under what circumstances).
- Step 4: Include any physicians' orders for side rail use.
- Step 5: Notify patient/resident and family of side rail use.
- Step 6: Obtain staff signatures and dates (include all members of the patient's/resident's interdisciplinary care team).

SAMPLE TOOL

A blank restraint assessment tool that can be used to compile this information is included in Part B of Section Two.

forms

performance-oriented environmental mobility screen (POEMS)

Instructions: Ask the patient or resident to perform the indicated maneuvers. If the individual uses an ambulation device (e.g., cane, walker), each maneuver is tested with the device as appropriate. For each maneuver, indicate whether the person's performance is normal (independent function) or impaired (dependent function). Suggested interventions for each impairment discovered (indicated by numbers in parentheses) are indicated. The key for the numbered interventions follows the forms.

Note: Each of the POEMS maneuvers has been printed on a separate page. The purpose of this design is to allow staff members to photocopy the POEMS and arrange the sequence of maneuvers according to their individual needs and those of patients or residents. In addition, the design allows for targeted assessments of risk (e.g., bed transfers, toilet transfers).

Falls in Older People: Prevention and Management, Third Edition,
by Rein Tideiksaar. Copyright © 2002, Health Professions Press, Inc., Baltimore.

Ambulation

Observation

Bedroom	Normal	Impaired (Intervention)
Walk in straight line from doorway to most distant wall (approx. 10–15 feet)	❑ Gait is continuous, without hesitation	❑ Gait is noncontinuous, with hesitation (1) (2)
	❑ Gait is straight, without deviation from path	❑ Gait deviates from straight path (1) (2) (5)
	❑ Both feet clear floor surface	❑ One or both feet scrape floor surface (1) (5) (6)
	❑ Does not use walls/furniture for support	❑ Walls/furniture are used for support (1) (2) (3) (4)
		❑ Unable to perform maneuver or perform it safely (10)
Turn around, walk around both sides of bed	❑ Steps are smooth, continuous	❑ Steps are discontinuous (1) (2) (5)
	❑ Does not stagger or lose balance	❑ Staggers, loses balance (1) (2) (5)
	❑ Does not use walls/furniture for support	❑ Walls/furniture are used for support (1) (2) (3) (4)
		❑ Unable to perform maneuver or perform it safely (10)
Device used to perform maneuver: ❑ Yes Type _____ ❑ No	❑ Device appropriate for space	❑ Device inappropriate for space (2) (4)
	❑ Device used correctly	❑ Device used incorrectly (2)

Falls in Older People: Prevention and Management, Third Edition,
by Rein Tideiksaar. Copyright © 2002, Health Professions Press, Inc., Baltimore.

Ambulation

	Observation	
Bathroom	Normal	Impaired (Intervention)
Walk to sink, toilet, turn around and return	❑ Gait is continuous, smooth without hesitation	❑ Gait is noncontinuous, with hesitation (1) (2)
	❑ Both feet clear floor and threshold	❑ One or both feet scrape floor or threshold (4) (5) (6)
	❑ Does not lose balance	❑ Loses balance (1) (2)
	❑ Does not use walls, sink, towel bar for balance support	❑ Uses walls, sink, towel bar for balance support (3) (4)
		❑ Unable to perform maneuver or perform it safely (10)
Device used to perform maneuver: ❑ Yes Type _____ ❑ No	❑ Device appropriate for space ❑ Device used correctly	❑ Device inappropriate for space (3) ❑ Device used incorrectly (2)

Ambulation

Observation

Hallway	Normal	Impaired (Intervention)
Walk from bedroom to nurses' station, toward exit, and return to bedroom	❏ Gait is continuous, without hesitation	❏ Gait is noncontinuous, with hesitation (1) (2) (5)
	❏ Gait is straight, without deviation from path	❏ Gait deviates from straight path (1) (2) (5)
	❏ Both feet clear floor surface	❏ One or both feet scrape floor surface (1) (5) (6)
	❏ Does not use walls/furniture/ handrails for support	❏ Walls/furniture/ handrails are used for support (1) (2) (3) (4)
	❏ Able to perform maneuver without excessive fatigue	❏ Unable to perform maneuver without fatigue (1) (10)
		❏ Unable to perform maneuver or perform it safely (10)
Device used to perform maneuver: ❏ Yes Type _____ ❏ No	❏ Device appropriate for space	❏ Device inappropriate for space (3)
	❏ Device used correctly	❏ Device used incorrectly (2)

Falls in Older People: Prevention and Management, Third Edition,
by Rein Tideiksaar. Copyright © 2002, Health Professions Press, Inc., Baltimore.

Transfers

	Observation	
Bed	**Normal**	**Impaired (Intervention)**
Transfer onto bed and lie down	❏ Bed transfer is completed in smooth, controlled movement (sits on bed in one attempt)	❏ Bed transfer is not smooth (requires several attempts; falls onto mattress; uses mattress edge to guide transfer) (1) (8)
	❏ Sitting balance is stable	❏ Sitting balance is unstable (2) (8)
	❏ Does not use arm support to maintain sitting balance	❏ Uses arm support to maintain sitting balance (2) (8)
	❏ Both feet rest flat on floor	❏ Feet do not rest flat on floor (8)
	❏ Feet do not slide	❏ Feet slide away (5) (6)
	❏ Bed does not slide away	❏ Bed slides away (6) (8)
	❏ Able to lie down in one smooth, controlled movement	❏ Unable to lie down in one smooth, controlled movement (several attempts required) (8)
		❏ Unable to perform maneuver or perform it safely (8) (10)
Device used to perform maneuver: ❏ Yes Type _____ ❏ No	❏ Device appropriate for space	❏ Device inappropriate for space (3)
	❏ Device used correctly	❏ Device used incorrectly (2)

(continued)

Transfers (bed—*continued*)

Bed	Normal	Impaired (Intervention)
Rise from supine position and transfer off bed	❑ Able to rise in one smooth, controlled movement to sitting position	❑ Unable to rise in one smooth, controlled movement to sitting position (several attempts required or cannot perform) (1) (8)
	❑ Sitting balance is stable	❑ Sitting balance is unstable (2) (8)
	❑ Does not use arm support to maintain sitting balance	❑ Uses arm support to maintain sitting balance (2) (8)
	❑ Both feet rest flat on floor	❑ Feet do not rest flat on floor (8)
	❑ Transfers off bed in smooth, controlled movement (rises off bed in one attempt)	❑ Transfer off bed is not completed in smooth, controlled movement (requires several attempts) (8)
	❑ Feet do not slide	❑ Feet slide away (5) (6)
	❑ Bed does not slide away	❑ Bed slides away (6) (8)
		❑ Unable to perform maneuver or perform it safely (8) (10)

Falls in Older People: Prevention and Management, Third Edition,
by Rein Tideiksaar. Copyright © 2002, Health Professions Press, Inc., Baltimore.

Transfers

Chair	Observation	
	Normal	Impaired (Intervention)
Sit down in chair(s)	❏ Sits in smooth, controlled movement (sits in one attempt)	❏ Sitting is not completed in smooth, controlled movement (requires several attempts) (1) (7)
	❏ Does not lose balance	❏ Loses balance (falls into seat) (2) (7)
	❏ Does not use arm rests for sitting	❏ Chair tips or slides away (7)
	❏ Chair does not tip or slide away	❏ Uses arm rests for sitting (7)
	❏ Seated, both feet rest flat on floor	❏ Seated, feet do not rest on floor (7)
		❏ Unable to perform maneuver or perform it safely (10)
Device used to perform maneuver: ❏ Yes Type _____ ❏ No	❏ Device appropriate for space ❏ Device used correctly	❏ Device inappropriate for space (2) (4) ❏ Device used incorrectly (2)

(continued)

Falls in Older People: Prevention and Management, Third Edition,
by Rein Tideiksaar. Copyright © 2002, Health Professions Press, Inc., Baltimore.

Transfers (chair—*continued*)

Chair	Normal	Impaired (Intervention)
Rises from chair	❑ Rises in smooth, controlled movement (rises in one attempt)	❑ Rising is not completed in smooth, controlled movement (requires several attempts) (1) (7)
	❑ Does not lose balance	❑ Loses balance (falls back into/off seat) (1) (7)
	❑ Does not use armrests	❑ Uses armrests or seat (7)
	❑ Chair does not tip or slide away	❑ Chair tips or slides away (7)
	❑ Feet do not slide on floor	❑ Feet slide on floor (5) (6) (7)
		❑ Unable to perform maneuver or perform it safely (10)

Falls in Older People: Prevention and Management, Third Edition,
by Rein Tideiksaar. Copyright © 2002, Health Professions Press, Inc., Baltimore.

Transfers

	Observation	
Toilet	Normal	Impaired (Intervention)
Sit down on toilet	❑ Able to sit down in one smooth, controlled movement	❑ Unable to sit down in one smooth, controlled movement (requires several attempts) (1) (9)
	❑ Does not lose balance	❑ Loses balance (1) (2) (9)
	❑ Does not use grab bars, sink edge for balance support	❑ Uses grab bars, sink edge for balance support (3) (4) (9)
	❑ Both feet rest flat on floor in seated position	❑ Feet do not rest flat on floor in seated position (9) (10)
		❑ Unable to perform maneuver or perform it safely (9) (10)
Device used to perform maneuver: ❑ Yes Type _____ ❑ No	❑ Device appropriate for space	❑ Device inappropriate for space (3)
	❑ Device used correctly	❑ Device used correctly (2)
Reach for toilet paper receptacle; simulate toilet hygiene	❑ Able to perform without excessive reach or balance loss	❑ Unable to perform without excessive reach or balance loss (9)
	❑ Does not use toilet, walls for balance support	❑ Uses toilet, walls for balance support (3) (9)
		❑ Unable to perform maneuver, or perform safely (10)

(continued)

Transfers *(toilet—continued)*

Toilet	Normal	Impaired (Intervention)
Rise from toilet	❑ Able to rise in one smooth, controlled movement	❑ Unable to rise in one smooth, controlled movement (requires several attempts) (1) (9)
	❑ Does not lose balance	❑ Loses balance (1) (3) (9)
	❑ Does not use grab bars, sink edge for balance support	❑ Uses grab bars, sink edge for balance support (3) (4) (9)
	❑ Feet do not slide away	❑ One or both feet slide away (5) (6)
		❑ Unable to perform maneuver or perform it safely (10)

Falls in Older People: Prevention and Management, Third Edition,
by Rein Tideiksaar. Copyright © 2002, Health Professions Press, Inc., Baltimore.

Balance

Observation

Standing/Reaching	Normal	Impaired (Intervention)
Stand in place (for approx. 15 seconds) with both eyes open	❏ Steady, able to stand without losing balance	❏ Unsteady, unable to maintain standing balance (1) (2)
	❏ Does not use chair to maintain balance	❏ Uses chair to maintain balance (7)
	❏ Does not use device to maintain balance	❏ Uses device to maintain balance (1) (2)
		❏ Unable to perform maneuver or perform it safely (10)
Stand in place with both eyes closed	❏ Steady, able to stand without losing balance	❏ Unsteady, unable to maintain standing balance (1) (2) (4)
	❏ Does not use chair to maintain balance	❏ Uses chair to maintain balance (7)
Stand in place (both eyes open); lightly nudge person's sternum 3 times	❏ Steady, able to maintain balance	❏ Unsteady, unable to maintain balance (1) (2)
	❏ Does not use furniture or walls to maintain balance	❏ Uses furniture or walls to maintain balance (7)
		❏ Unable to perform maneuver or perform it safely (10)
Bend down and pick up object from floor	❏ Steady, able to bend down without losing balance	❏ Unsteady, unable to bend down and maintain balance (1)

(continued)

Falls in Older People: Prevention and Management, Third Edition,
by Rein Tideiksaar. Copyright © 2002, Health Professions Press, Inc., Baltimore.

Balance (standing/reaching—*continued*)

Standing/Reaching	Normal	Impaired (Intervention)
	❑ Does not use device to maintain balance	❑ Uses device to maintain balance (1) (2) ❑ Unable to perform maneuver or perform it safely (10)

Key to Interventions

1. Medical evaluation
2. Rehabilitative evaluation
   - ❑ Nonslip strips
   - ❑ Gait assessment
   - ❑ Balance assessment
   - ❑ Exercise program
   - ❑ Hip-padding system
   - ❑ Other: _____
3. Walking space/pathways
   - ❑ Unobstructed walking areas
   - ❑ Stable furnishings for support
   - ❑ Nonslip grasp surfaces (furnishings, walls, sink, hallways)
   - ❑ Other: _____
4. Visual walking space/pathways
   - ❑ Accessible lighting
   - ❑ Adequate lighting
   - ❑ Glare reduction
   - ❑ Color contrast (furnishings, handrails, grab bars)
   - ❑ Other: _____
5. Footwear
   - ❑ Podiatrist evaluation
   - ❑ Proper fit
   - ❑ Nonslip soles/socks
   - ❑ Nontraction soles
   - ❑ Other: _____
6. Floor space
   - ❑ Nonslip finishes
   - ❑ Nonslip strips
   - ❑ Eliminate uneven surface elevations
   - ❑ Color contrast uneven surface elevations
   - ❑ Other: _____

7. Chair
   - ❑ Seat height adjustment
   - ❑ Seat depth adjustment
   - ❑ Supportive armrests
   - ❑ Stable (nonmovable) chair
   - ❑ Seat cushions/wedge cushion
   - ❑ Other: _____
8. Bed
   - ❑ Height adjustment (low/high)
   - ❑ Firm mattress support
   - ❑ Bed half side rail
   - ❑ Transfer bar
   - ❑ Bed wheel locks
   - ❑ Immobilizer legs
   - ❑ Bed alarm device
   - ❑ Accessible nurse call system
   - ❑ Other: _____
9. Toilet
   - ❑ Grab bar (wall/toilet attached)
   - ❑ Raised toilet seat
   - ❑ Accessible nurse call system
   - ❑ Bedside commode
   - ❑ Other: _____
10. Human assistance
    - ❑ One person
    - ❑ Two people
    - ❑ Other: _____

POEMS Summary

Location	Maneuver	Normal	Impaired
Bedroom	Ambulation		
	Straight line	❑	❑
	Turning	❑	❑
	Chair transfer		
	Onto	❑	❑
	Off	❑	❑
	Standing balance		
	Eyes open	❑	❑
	Eyes closed	❑	❑
	Sternal nudge	❑	❑
	Bending down	❑	❑
	Bed transfer		
	Onto	❑	❑
	Off	❑	❑
Bathroom	Ambulation		
	Straight line	❑	❑
	Turning	❑	❑
	Toilet transfer		
	Onto	❑	❑
	Off	❑	❑
	Toilet hygiene	❑	❑
Hallway	Ambulation		
	Straight line	❑	❑
	Turning	❑	❑
	Distance	❑	❑

Falls in Older People: Prevention and Management, Third Edition,
by Rein Tideiksaar. Copyright © 2002, Health Professions Press, Inc., Baltimore.

Injury and Acute Medical Problems Checklist

Summon for medical assistance if patient/resident complains of

	Yes	No
Difficulty moving arms or legs?	❏	❏
Pain/injury in arms, legs, or lower back?	❏	❏
Headache/head injury?	❏	❏
Confusion/lethargy?	❏	❏
Dizziness/lightheadedness?	❏	❏
Loss of consciousness?	❏	❏
Convulsions?	❏	❏
Chest pain/difficulty breathing?	❏	❏
Fast, slow, or irregular pulse rate?	❏	❏

If you suspect a hip or pelvic fracture (e.g., pain in hip, lower back, or groin area; extremity pain that worsens with movement), do not try to move the person.

Falls in Older People: Prevention and Management, Third Edition,
by Rein Tideiksaar. Copyright © 2002, Health Professions Press, Inc., Baltimore.

Fall Risk Checklist

Risk factors

- ❏ Previous falls
- ❏ Visual impairment
- ❏ Postural hypotension
- ❏ Balance disorder
- ❏ Cognitive impairment
  (depression, dementia,
  poor judgment)
- ❏ Gait disorder

- ❏ Lower extremity weakness
- ❏ Arthritis (knee, hips)
- ❏ Medications (psychotropics,
  sedatives, hypnotics,
  antihypertensives)
- ❏ Bladder and/or bowel dysfunction
  (frequency, urgency, nocturia,
  incontinence)

Describe circumstances of falls
Symptoms:

Location:

Time of day:

Activity:

Trauma:

Mobility

Location	Maneuver	Independent	Impaired
Bedroom	Chair transfers		
	Sitting	❏	❏
	Rising	❏	❏
	Standing balance	❏	❏
	Immediate	❏	❏
	Romberg test	❏	❏
	Sternal push test	❏	❏
	Bending-down balance	❏	❏
	Bed transfers		
	Sitting	❏	❏
	Rising	❏	❏
	Ambulation		
	Straight path	❏	❏
	Turning	❏	❏
Bathroom	Toilet transfers		
	Sitting	❏	❏
	Rising	❏	❏
	Ambulation		
	Straight path	❏	❏
	Turning	❏	❏
	Other	❏	❏

_____

_____

Restraint/Non-Restraint Assessment and Care Planning Tool

Date: _____

[Patient's/resident's name]

PART I: Baseline Patient/Resident Information

Does the patient/resident:	Yes	No
Have poor judgment or impaired communication?	❏	❏
Have a history of recent falls?	❏	❏
Have contractures or limited range of motion?	❏	❏
Have difficulty with postural hypotension?	❏	❏
Have a diagnosis of or signs and symptoms of depression?	❏	❏
Have difficulty with standing/sitting balance?	❏	❏
Have a history of wandering?	❏	❏

Is the patient/resident:		
Able to toilet independently?	❏	❏
On any medications requiring safety precautions?	❏	❏
Able to use the call light?	❏	❏
Continent?	❏	❏
Agitated?	❏	❏
Interfering with his or her medical treatment?	❏	❏

PART II: Describe the patient's/resident's medical, psychological, and functional problems indicating potential need for restraint use.

PART III: Nonrestraint justification. Describe the care plan (including non-restraint alternatives) provided to patient/resident and why nonrestraint is being considered at this time. Consider

Low beds

Mats on floor

Half-side rails as enablers

Bed alarms

Wedge cushions/other positioning devices

Moving patient/resident nearer to nurses' station

Fall prevention program

Falls in Older People: Prevention and Management, Third Edition,
by Rein Tideiksaar. Copyright © 2002, Health Professions Press, Inc., Baltimore.

(continued)

PART IV: Restraint use justification. Describe the care plan (including least-restraint/restraint-alternative efforts to date) provided to the patient/resident and why restraint is being considered at this time.

PART V: Describe the restraint recommendations (including restraint-monitoring schedule).

PART VI: Physician's order for restraint.

Does the order include the following:

	Yes	No
Specific type of restraint used?	❏	❏
The circumstances or conditions under which the restraint should be used?	❏	❏
Restraint release/reduction times?	❏	❏

PART VII: Patient/resident and family notification of restraint/non-restraint recommendations

I understand why the interdisciplinary team has recommended restraints/non-restraints as part of [patient's/resident's name] care plan. I am aware certain negative outcomes such as falls are associated with [restraint/non-restraint] use.

❏ Approve

❏ Disapprove

Signature: _____ Date: _____
           Family representative or legal guardian

Signature: _____ Date: _____
                    Patient/resident

(continued)

PART VIII: Staff signatures (include all members of the patient's/resident's interdisciplinary care team)

Side Rail Assessment and Care Planning Tool

Date: _____

Patient's/resident's name: _____

PART I: Baseline Assessment Information

Is the patient/resident:	Yes	No
Ambulatory (including assistive devices)?	❑	❑
Comatose, semi-comatose, or having fluctuations in mental status?	❑	❑
Able to toilet independently?	❑	❑
Able to transfer from bed independently?	❑	❑
Able to ambulate to the bathroom (toilet) independently?	❑	❑
Continent?	❑	❑
On any medications that would require increased safety precautions?	❑	❑

Does the patient/resident:		
Have poor judgment or impaired communication?	❑	❑
Have a diagnosis or symptoms of depression?	❑	❑
Have falls from bed?	❑	❑
Have falls on the way to bathroom (toilet)?	❑	❑
Have postural hypotension?	❑	❑
Have contractures or limited range of motion?	❑	❑

Falls in Older People: Prevention and Management, Third Edition,
by Rein Tideiksaar. Copyright © 2002, Health Professions Press, Inc., Baltimore.

(continued)

Side Rail Assessment and Care Planning Tool *(continued)*

PART II: Describe rationale for potential side rail use.

Include the following:

	Yes	No
Patient/resident has requested to have side rail raised while in bed.	❏	❏
Side rails serve as:		
An enabler to promote mobility while in bed	❏	❏
An enabler to promote safe bed transfers	❏	❏
Side rails are indicated to provide safety or prevent falls at this time. (If yes, explain why.)	❏	❏

PART III: Side rail use recommendations. Describe when and why side rails are used (i.e., how long and under what circumstances).

Falls in Older People: Prevention and Management, Third Edition,
by Rein Tideiksaar. Copyright © 2002, Health Professions Press, Inc., Baltimore.

PART IV: Physician's order for side rail use. Does the order include the following:

	Yes	No
Specific type of side rail?	❏	❏
Under what circumstances or conditions side rails are used?	❏	❏
Side rail monitoring times?	❏	❏

PART V: Patient/resident and family notification of side rail use

I understand why the interdisciplinary team has recommended side rails as part of (patient's/resident's name) care plan. I am aware that certain negative outcomes are associated with side rail use.

❏ Approve

❏ Disapprove

Signature: _____ Date: _____
                       Family representative or legal guardian

Signature: _____ Date: _____
                            Patient/resident

PART VI: Staff signatures and dates (include all members of the patient's/resident's interdisciplinary care team)

Wheelchair Problems and Modifications Checklist

Observe patients' or residents' wheelchair mobility. Ask each individual to transfer from the chair and observe whether he or she accomplishes the task safely.

	Yes	No
Did the person engage the brakes?	❑	❑

If no, consider wedge cushion to prevent independent transfers.

	Yes	No
Can the person reach the hand brakes?	❑	❑

If no, replace with long brake handles.

	Yes	No
Did the brakes lock in place?	❑	❑

If no, replace the chair or fix the problem.

	Yes	No
Did the person remember to move the footrests away?	❑	❑

If no, consider removing footrests (if appropriate) or consider adding a wedge cushion to prevent independent transfers.

	Yes	No
Did the chair tip over forward?	❑	❑

If yes, consider attaching antitip device to footplates or weights to the back of the chair.

	Yes	No
Does the seat interfere with transfers?	❑	❑

If yes, consider retrofitting sling seat with plywood or solid inserts.

	Yes	No
Does the seat interfere with sitting balance?	❑	❑

If yes, consider lateral supports to correct lean.

	Yes	No
Does individual slide out of chair seat?	❑	❑

If yes, consider use of Dycem mat (placed on seat to prevent sliding) or position footrests to maintain proper seating.

discharge teaching sheets

Home Fall Prevention

An injury from falling can limit a person's ability to lead an active, independent life. This is especially true for older people. Each year, thousands of older men and women are injured, sometimes permanently, by falls that result in broken bones. Yet many of these injuries can be prevented by making simple changes in the home.

As people age, changes in their vision, hearing, muscle strength, coordination, and reflexes may make them susceptible to falls. Older adults likely have treatable disorders that may affect their balance (e.g., diabetes; conditions of the heart, nervous system, and thyroid). In addition, as compared with younger adults, older people often take medications that may cause dizziness or lightheadedness.

Preventing falls is especially important for people with osteoporosis, a condition in which bone mass decreases so that bones are more fragile and break easily. Osteoporosis is a major cause of bone fractures in women after menopause and older adults in general. For people with severe osteoporosis, even a minor fall may cause one or more bones to break.

STEPS TO TAKE

Falls and accidents seldom "just happen," and many can be prevented. Each of us can take steps to make our homes safer and

Falls in Older People: Prevention and Management, Third Edition,
by Rein Tideiksaar. Copyright © 2002, Health Professions Press, Inc., Baltimore.

reduce the likelihood of falling. Here are some guidelines to help prevent falls and fractures:

- Vision and hearing should be tested regularly and properly corrected.
- The person should talk with the doctor or pharmacist about the side effects of the medicines he or she is taking and whether they affect coordination or balance. The person should ask for suggestions to reduce the possibility of falling.
- The person should limit his or her alcohol intake. Even a small amount of alcohol can disturb already-impaired balance and reflexes.
- The person should use caution in getting up too quickly after eating, lying down, or resting. Low blood pressure may cause dizziness at these times.
- The nighttime temperature in the person's home should be at least 65°F. Prolonged exposure to cold temperatures may cause a drop in body temperature, which in turn may lead to dizziness and falling. Many older adults cannot tolerate cold as well as younger people can.
- A cane, a walking stick, or a walker should be used to help the person maintain balance on uneven or unfamiliar ground or if the person sometimes feels dizzy. Special caution should be taken in walking outdoors on wet or icy pavement.
- The person should wear supportive rubber-soled or low-heeled shoes and avoid wearing smooth-soled slippers or socks without shoes on stairs and waxed floors. These surfaces make it easy to slip.
- The person should maintain a regular program of exercise to improve strength and muscle tone, and joints, tendons, and ligaments should be kept flexible. Many older people enjoy walking and swimming. Mild weight-bearing activities, such as walking or climbing stairs, may even reduce bone loss due to osteoporosis. The person should check with his or her doctor or physical therapist to plan a suitable exercise program.

Falls in Older People: Prevention and Management, Third Edition,
by Rein Tideiksaar. Copyright © 2002, Health Professions Press, Inc., Baltimore.

MAKE HOME A SAFE PLACE

Many older people fall because of hazardous conditions at home. This checklist can be used to help safeguard the person against some likely hazards.

Stairways, hallways, and pathways should have

☐ Good lighting. Provide extra lighting along path from bedroom to bathroom, by one- and two-step elevations, and by top and bottom of stairway landings; use night-light, 100- to 200-watt bulbs, and 3-way lightbulbs to increase lighting levels

☐ A lack of glare. Eliminate glare from exposed lightbulbs by using translucent light shades or frosted lightbulbs.

☐ Firmly attached carpet, rough-texture or abrasive strips to secure footing, nonskid rugs and carpet runners on slippery floors, a coating of nonskid floor wax, carpeting over threshold to create a smooth transition between rooms

☐ No clutter, including obtrusive furnishings

☐ Tightly fastened cylindrical handrails running the whole length and along both sides of all stairs, with light switches at the top and bottom

Bathrooms should have

☐ Elevated toilet seat or toilet safety frame

☐ Wall-mounted or tub-attached grab bar or shower chair/tub transfer bench

☐ Nonskid mats, abrasive strips, or carpet on all surfaces that may get wet

☐ Night-lights

Bedrooms should have

☐ Night-lights or light switches within reach of bed(s)

☐ Telephones that are easy to reach near the bed(s)

Falls in Older People: Prevention and Management, Third Edition,
by Rein Tideiksaar. Copyright © 2002, Health Professions Press, Inc., Baltimore.

Living areas should have

- ❏ Electrical cords and telephone wires placed away from walking paths
- ❏ Rugs well secured to the floor
- ❏ Furniture, especially low coffee tables, and other objects arranged so that they are not obstacles
- ❏ Couches and chairs that are of a proper height so that patients or residents get into and out of them easily (add a seat cushion to raise seat height; replace existing mattress with one that is thinner to lower bed height, or thicker to raise bed height); chairs with armrest support
- ❏ Frequently used objects sited at waist level
- ❏ A reacher device available for person to obtain objects from shelves
- ❏ Shelves and cupboards at accessible height

appendix

case study exercises

CASE 1

E.L. is an 80-year-old hospital patient who experienced two falls. She stated that both falls occurred shortly after she got up from bed at night to go to the bathroom. She was hurrying to the toilet in order to avoid urinating on the floor and lost her balance. Her medical problems consist of Parkinson's disease and arthritis in both knees. She takes no medication. E.L.'s ambulation is poor and she does not use a walker. Her cognitive abilities are unaffected.

Questions

1. With the information you have about this patient, what specific interventions would you include in her care plan in order to reduce fall risk?
2. Based on your care plan, for which outcomes would you monitor this patient?

CASE 2

G.B. is a 76-year-old nursing facility resident who experienced several falls from bed. He complained of unsteadiness after getting up from bed. G.B.'s medical problems include a history of hypertension, which was treated with a diuretic. The results of the medical evaluation revealed that G.B. was dehydrated and had orthostatic hypotension (i.e., dizziness on rising from a seated or lying position).

Questions

1. With the information you have about this resident, what specific interventions would you include in his care plan in order to reduce fall risk?

2. Based on your care plan, for which outcomes would you monitor this resident?

CASE 3

M.P. is an 89-year-old nursing facility resident who experienced several falls, all of which occurred while she was walking either in the bedroom or hallway in the late afternoon. M.P.'s medical problem consists of severe dementia. She exhibits poor gait and balance. M.P. has a walker but forgets to use it. Since her original diagnosis, M.P.'s cognition has deteriorated further, resulting in agitation. M.P. does not take medication.

Questions

1. With the information you have about this resident, what specific interventions would you include in her care plan in order to reduce fall risk?
2. Based on your care plan, for which outcomes would you monitor this resident?

CASE 4

J.S. is an 82-year-old hospital patient who was admitted for pneumonia. He remained in bed for 3 days. After treatment of the illness, the patient demonstrated poor bed and toilet transfers, which was the result of lower-leg weakness developed after being confined to bed.

Questions

1. With the information you have about this patient, what specific interventions would you include in his care plan in order to improve mobility and reduce fall risk?
2. Based on your care plan, for which outcomes would you monitor this patient?

CASE 5

L.R. is a 73-year-old hospital patient admitted for falls. After her most recent fall, she lay on the floor unattended for 6 hours (she lives alone). L.R.'s falls are associated with a loss of balance—which she experiences when she reaches up to retrieve objects from her kitchen and closet shelves and when she gets into and out of her bathtub. L.R. has experienced a stroke and, as a result, has mild left-side leg weakness. She expresses a fear of falling.

Questions

1. With the information you have about this patient, what specific interventions would you include in her care plan in order to improve mobility and reduce her fear of falls while she is in the hospital?
2. What specific interventions would you include in her postdischarge care plan?

CASE 6

A.C. is a 91-year-old nursing facility resident who has experienced several falls from his wheelchair. His falls occur as he attempts to transfer onto his bed and toilet. In a few instances he has slid out of his wheelchair and onto the floor; on one occasion his wheelchair tipped over during a transfer. A.C.'s medical history includes a stroke with associated leg weakness and depression for which he takes an antidepressant. Occasionally, he feels dizzy when transferring from his wheelchair.

Questions

1. With the information you have about this resident, what specific interventions would you include in his care plan in order to decrease the risk of falls from his wheelchair?
2. Based on your care plan, for which outcomes would you monitor this resident?

CASE 7

R.E. is an 89-year-old nursing facility resident with moderate dementia, arthritis of the knees, and polymyalgia rheumatica (i.e., a syndrome affecting older people characterized by proximal joint or muscle pain) for which he takes steroid medication. He demonstrates poor bed transfers and ambulation. R.E. uses a walker, but the device is unsafe.

Questions

1. With the information you have about this resident, what specific interventions would you include in his care plan in order to reduce fall risk?
2. Based on your care plan, for which outcomes would you monitor this resident?

CASE 8

M.S. is an 82-year-old hospital patient admitted for falls. She demonstrates poor bed, toilet, and chair transfers, which are the result of lower limb weakness. M.S.'s cognition is mildly impaired. She has hypothyroidism and is on replacement therapy.

Questions

1. With the information you have about this patient, what specific interventions would you include in her care plan in order to improve mobility and reduce fall risk?
2. Based on your care plan, for which outcomes would you monitor this patient?

CASE 9

W.M. is a 79-year-old hospital patient. On the day she was admitted, she slipped in her urine while attempting to toilet. W.M. is now afraid to go to the bathroom by herself and has developed a fear of falling. As a result of this fear, she has developed urinary incontinence. She is able to transfer independently and her cognitive abilities are unaffected.

Questions

1. With the information you have about this patient, what specific intervention would you include in her care plan in order to reduce incontinence and her fear of falling?
2. Based on your care plan, for which outcomes would you monitor this patient?

CASE 10

M.M. is an 82-year-old nursing facility resident who has experienced several falls from bed. M.M.'s medical problems consist of Parkinson's disease and osteoporosis. She takes no medication. Recently, her nurses found M.M. sprawled on the floor by her bed. To prevent further bed falls she was placed in mechanical restraints.

Questions

1. With the information you have about this resident, what specific interventions would you include in her care plan to reduce the risk of falls and eliminate the need for mechanical restraints?
2. Based on your care plan, for which outcomes would you monitor this resident?

CASE 11

L.B. is a 76-year-old woman admitted to the hospital emergency room following a left-sided cerebrovascular accident (CVA) with aphasia. After 2 days, she was transferred to the rehabilitation unit for treatment.

Questions

1. With the information you have about this patient, what specific interventions would you include in her care plan in order to reduce fall risk?
2. Based on your care plan, for which outcomes would you monitor this patient?

CASE 12

T.S. is a 95-year-old man with Parkinson's disease. His nursing aide notices that T.S. has difficulty getting up from his bed. Until now, the patient's bed transfers have been normal.

Questions

1. With the information you have about this patient, what specific interventions would you include in his care plan in order to reduce fall risk?

2. Based on your care plan, for which outcomes would you monitor this patient?

CASE 13

S.O. is a 72-year-old nursing facility resident with confusion. She experienced a fall while walking to the bathroom.

Questions

1. With the information you have about this patient, what specific interventions would you include in her care plan in order to reduce fall risk?
2. Based on your care plan, for which outcomes would you monitor this resident?

CASE 14

A.S. is an 84-year-old hospital patient with diabetes and arthritis. He experiences gait and balance impairment but doesn't use his walker.

Questions

1. With the information you have about this patient, what specific interventions would you include in his care plan in order to reduce fall risk?
2. Based on your care plan, for which outcomes would you monitor this patient?

CASE 15

P.P. is an 88-year-old nursing facility resident. She has experienced two falls while getting up from an easy chair located in her bedroom. Now she has a fear of falling.

Questions

1. With the information you have about this resident, what specific interventions would you include in her care plan in order to reduce fall risk?

2. Based on your care plan, for which outcomes would you monitor this resident?

CASE 16

I.S. is a 71-year-old man admitted to the hospital for elective total knee arthroplasty for severe degenerative joint disease that has led to a decline in function and increasing pain. On the evening of the second hospital day, I.S. began to exhibit some confusion.

Questions

1. With the information you have about this resident, what specific interventions would you include in his care plan in order to reduce fall risk?
2. Based on your care plan, for which outcomes would you monitor this patient?

Answers for Case 1

Question 1

- Primary care provider to evaluate patient's nocturia (i.e., getting up at night to urinate) for reversible causes.
- Primary care provider to evaluate patient's Parkinson's disease and arthritis and her need for Parkinson's and analgesic medications in order to improve ambulation.
- Nursing to provide a night-light in patient's bedroom in order to provide safe ambulation to the bathroom.
- Physical Therapy to evaluate patient for a walker in order to improve ambulation.
- Physical Therapy to evaluate patient and provide an exercise program in order to improve ambulation.

Question 2

- Monitor patient for further falls. If falls occur under similar circumstances, consider a bed alarm system to alert staff when E.L. gets out of bed and so that they can offer assistance with ambulation, or provide a bedside commode to eliminate E.L.'s need to travel to the bathroom.
- Monitor symptoms of nocturia.
- Monitor patient's ability to ambulate and for safe use of her walker.

Answers for Case 2

Question 1

- Primary care provider to evaluate the dose of diuretic in order to reduce risk of dehydration and orthostatic hypotension.
- Nursing to provide resident with sufficient fluid intake in order to treat dehydration.
- Nursing to request that resident asks for assistance when getting up from bed and to provide assistance with rising from bed in order to reduce risk of falls.
- Nursing to check whether resident also experiences orthostatic hypotension with other transfer activities, such as chair and toilet transfers, and provide appropriate modifications as needed in order to support safe transfer activities.

Question 2

- Monitor G.B. for further falls. If falls occur, refer to primary care provider for another evaluation. If falls occur with rising from bed or resident fails to ask for assistance, or both, consider the use of a bed alarm system.
- Monitor G.B.'s blood pressure to ensure that it is controlled, particularly if the dose of diuretics is reduced.
- Monitor fluid intake to avoid the risk of dehydration.

Answers for Case 3

Question 1

- Primary care provider to evaluate resident's worsening cognition and agitation for reversible causes. Consider short-term medication to control agitation, but only if behavior results in harm to self or others.
- Physical Therapy to evaluate resident and provide a walker and an ambulation program in order to support safe ambulation.
- Nursing to provide resident with structured activities in the late afternoon in order to avoid agitation and eliminate need for medication to control agitation.

Question 2

- Monitor for further falls. If falls occur under similar circumstances, consider hip-padding system in order to decrease risk of hip fractures.
- Monitor cognition and agitation.

- Monitor for effectiveness and side effects of medication, if given for agitation.
- Monitor ambulation and for safe use of walker. If resident fails to use her walker, consider a Merry Walker to allow independent ambulation.
- Monitor for sundowning (i.e., late afternoon or early evening confusion).

Answers for Case 4

Question 1

- Primary care provider to evaluate patient's leg weakness for treatable causes.
- Physical Therapy to evaluate patient and provide rehabilitative exercise program to improve his leg strength.
- Nursing to evaluate patient's bed and provide modifications such as low height, half bed side rail for transfer assistance, and nonslip floor surfaces in order to support safe transfers.
- Physical Therapy to evaluate patient's toilet and provide modifications such as grab bars, toilet riser, and nonslip floor surface in order to support safe transfers.
- Nursing to request that patient asks for help with transfers and to provide assistance in order to support safe transfers.

Question 2

- Monitor patient for further falls. If patient falls from bed, fails to ask for assistance, or both, consider bed alarm system to alert staff when patient gets out of bed.
- Monitor for effectiveness of bed and toilet modifications.
- Monitor for effectiveness of rehabilitative exercise program.

Answers for Case 5

Question 1

- Primary care provider to evaluate the causes of the patient's falls and risk factors for further falls (i.e., to examine for treatable causes and modifiable risk factors).
- Physical Therapy to evaluate patient and provide an exercise program in order to improve L.P.'s balance and reduce her fear of falling.
- Nursing to provide assistance with patient's transfers and ambulation in order to support safe activities and reduce her fear of falling.

Question 2

- Home Care to provide patient with a personal emergency response system in order to reduce the risk of extensive lie times.
- Home Care Physical Therapy to continue exercise program, if needed.
- Home Care Occupational Therapy to evaluate the safety of L.P.'s home environment; modify kitchen/closet shelves in order to reduce risk of balance loss and provide bathtub equipment in order to support safe tub transfers.

Answers for Case 6

Question 1

- Primary care provider to evaluate resident's depression and antidepressant dosage for medication side effects and possible decreased medication dose or selection of an alternative drug.
- Physical Therapy to teach resident safe wheelchair transfer techniques, provide an exercise program to strengthen his legs, modify resident's wheelchair (e.g., brakes, seat height, and anti-tipping device to support safe transfers), and provide toilet grab bars and half bed side rail to support safe toilet and bed transfers.
- Nursing to provide resident with a nonslip wheelchair seat cushion in order to prevent him from sliding out of his wheelchair.

Question 2

- Monitor for further falls from the wheelchair. If falls occur, reevaluate wheelchair interventions.
- Monitor depression and effectiveness/side effects of medication.
- Monitor for effectiveness of Physical Therapy and Nursing interventions.

Answers for Case 7

Question 1

- Primary care provider to evaluate resident's steroid medication for necessity or for tapering off of the dosage.
- Nursing to evaluate resident's bed and provide modifications, such as lower height and half bed side rails, for transfer assistance to support safe transfers.
- Physical Therapy to evaluate resident's walker and the need for an exercise program in order to improve leg strength and ambulation.

Question 2

* Monitor for further falls from bed.
* Monitor bed transfers and for effectiveness of bed modifications.
* Monitor ambulation and for safe use of the walker.

Answers for Case 8

Question 1

* Primary care provider to evaluate patient's leg weakness and altered cognition for treatable causes.
* Nursing to evaluate patient's bed and provide modifications in order to support safe transfers.
* Physical Therapy to evaluate patient and provide an exercise program in order to improve transfers. PT to evaluate and provide chair and toilet modifications in order to support safe transfers.

Question 2

* Monitor for further falls.
* Monitor thyroid status and for effectiveness of replacement therapy.
* Monitor cognition.
* Monitor transfers.
* Monitor for effectiveness of chair and toilet modifications.

Answers for Case 9

Question 1

* Nursing to provide patient with a bedside commode to eliminate the need for traveling to the bathroom and to reduce incontinence.
* Nursing to provide assistance with toileting, as needed.
* Nonslip strips of a noncontrasting color to be applied to patient's bathroom floor in the event that patient resumes bathroom activity.

Question 2

* Monitor for incontinence.
* Monitor for fear of falling.
* Monitor for effectiveness of bedside commode.

Answers for Case 10

Question 1

• Primary care provider to evaluate resident's Parkinson's disease for the need for medication.

• Nursing to evaluate resident's bed and provide modifications in order to support safe bed transfers. Mechanical restraints to be removed from the resident. If the resident continues to fall, consider the use of a bed alarm system.

• Nursing to evaluate resident's need for low-height bed to reduce the risk of injurious falls from bed. Provide bed, if necessary.

Question 2

• Monitor for further falls from bed.

• Monitor Parkinson's disease and for effectiveness of medications, if given.

• Monitor for effectiveness of bed alarm system, if used.

• Monitor for effectiveness of low-height bed, if used.

Answers for Case 11

Question 1

• Physical Therapy to evaluate patient's mobility and transfers, and an ambulation device (e.g., walker).

• Nursing to evaluate patient's risk of falling.

• Nursing to evaluate patient's communication (e.g., ability to use nurse call bell and request assistance).

Question 2

• Monitor mobility and bed transfers.

• Monitor ambulation and safe use of walker.

• Monitor use of call bell and consider a bed alarm system if patient is noncompliant.

• Monitor risk of falling and reassess risk as patient's condition improves.

Answers to Case 12

Question 1

• Nursing to evaluate patient's immediate risk for bed falls.

• Nursing to consider lowering bed height and/or using siderail as enabling device to support safe bed transfers.

- Physical Therapy to evaluate patient's mobility and transfers.
- Physician to evaluate patient's change of condition.
- Nursing aide to observe patient's bed transfers every shift.

Question 2

- Monitor bed transfers and safety interventions established. If patient continues to experience impaired bed transfers, consider using side rail as enabling device to support bed transfers.

Answers to Case 13

Question 1

- Nursing to review circumstances of resident's fall.
- Nursing to reassess resident's risk for falls.
- Nursing to communicate resident's risk status to other staff members.
- Physician to evaluate resident's cognitive status and cause of confusion.
- Physical Therapy to evaluate resident's gait and balance.
- Nursing to provide resident with daily ambulation assistance, as needed.

Question 2

- Monitor resident's ambulation status.
- Monitor resident's cognitive status.
- Monitor resident's risk for falls.
- Monitor resident for change of condition.

Answers to Case 14

Question 1

- Physician to evaluate patient's medical conditions and need for disease management.
- Physical Therapy to evaluate patient's mobility and appropriateness of walker.
- Physical Therapy to evaluate patient for exercises to improve gait and balance.
- Nursing to evaluate patient for assistance with ambulation needs.

Question 2

- Monitor patient's diabetes and arthritis.
- Monitor patient's gait and balance.
- Monitor patient's compliance with walker.

Answers to Case 15

Question 1

- Nursing to provide safety with resident's chair transfers (e.g., need for assistance with transfers or replace chair with one that the resident is able to transfer safely from).
- Nursing to evaluate resident's fear of falling (i.e., has her concern about falling restricted her mobility?).
- Physician to evaluate resident for change of condition.
- Physical Therapy to evaluate resident's chair transfers and need for chair modifications.

Question 2

- Monitor resident's chair transfers.
- Monitor resident's risk for further falls.
- Monitor resident's fear of falling and provide assistance with mobility until resident regains confidence.

Answers to Case 16

Question 1

- Physician to evaluate for causes of patient's confusion and pain.
- Nursing to evaluate patient's risk for falls with condition change and safety interventions as needed.
- Physical Therapy to evaluate patient's functional status and needs.

Question 2

- Monitor patient's mental status.
- Monitor patient's pain.
- Monitor patient's functional status.
- Monitor patient's risk for falls.

bibliography

An asterisk following a reference indicates a reference covering fall-risk assessment tools.

HOSPITAL

Aisen, P.S., Deluca, T., & Lawlor, B.A. (1992). Falls among geropsychiatry inpatients are associated with PRN medications for agitation. *International Journal of Geriatric Psychiatry, 7*, 709–712.

Ashton, J., Gilbert, D., Hayward, G., et al. (1989). Predicting patient falls in an acute care setting. *Kansas Nurse, 64*(10), 3–5.

Baker, L. (1992). Developing a safety plan that works for patients and nurses. *Rehabilitation Nursing, 17*, 264–266.

Bates, D.W., Pruess, K., Souney, P., & Platt, R. (1995). Serious falls in hospitalized patients: Correlates and resource utilization. *American Journal of Medicine, 99*, 137–143.

Berryman, E., Gaskin, D., Jones, A., et al. (1989, July/August). Point by point: Predicting elders' falls. *Geriatric Nursing*, 199–201.*

Brady, R., Cheater, F.R., Pierce, L.L., et al. (1993). Geriatric falls: Prevention strategies for the staff. *Journal of Gerontological Nursing, 19*, 26–32.

Brians, L.K., Alexander, K., Grota, P., et al. (1991). The development of the RISK tool for fall prevention. *Rehabilitation Nursing, 16*(2), 67–69.*

Burden, B., & Kishi, D. (1989). Patient falls: lowering the risk. *Nursing, 16*(2), 79.*

Byers, V., Arrington, M.E., & Finstuen, K. (1990). Predictive risk factors associated with stroke patient falls in acute care settings. *Journal of Neuroscience Nursing, 22*(3), 147–154.

Caley, L.M., & Pinchoff, D.M. (1994). A comparison study of patient falls in a psychiatric setting. *Hospital and Community Psychiatry, 45*, 823–825.

Chu, L.W., Pei, C.K., Chiu, A., Liu, K., Chu, M.M., Wong, S., & Wong, A. (1999). Risk factors for falls in hospitalized older medical patients. *Journal of Gerontology, 54*, M38–M43.

Cohen, L., & Guin, P. (1991). Implementation of a patient fall prevention program. *Journal of Neuroscience Nursing, 23*(5), 315–319.

Commodore, D.I. (1995). Falls in the elderly population: A look at incidence, risks, healthcare costs, and preventive strategies. *Rehabilitation Nursing, 20*(2), 84–89.

Corbett, C., & Pennypacker, B. (1992). Using a quality improvement team to reduce patient falls. *Journal of Hospital Quality, 14*, 38–54.*

Dallaire, L.B., & Burke, E.V. (1989). Reducing patient falls. *Nursing, 19* (1), 65.

de Carle, A.J., & Kohn, R. (2001). Risk factors for falling in a psychogeriatric unit. *International Journal of Geriatric Psychiatry, 16*, 762–767.

Easterling, M.L. (1990). Which of your patients is headed for a fall? *RN, 53* (1), 56–59.

Evans, D., Hodgkinson, B., Lambert, L., & Wood, J. (2001). Fall risk factors in the hospital setting: A systematic review. *International Journal of Nursing Practice, 7*, 38–45.

Fleck, M.M., & Forrester, D.A. (2001). The efficacy of an education program to improve direct caregiver knowledge regarding fall prevention. *Journal for Nurses in Staff Development, 17*, 27–33.

Gaebler, S. (1993). Predicting which patient will fall again . . . and again. *Journal of Advanced Nursing, 18*, 1895–1902.

Goodwin, M.B., & Westbrook, J.I. (1993). An analysis of patient accidents in hospital. *Australian Clinical Review, 13*, 141–149.

Greene, E., Cunningham, C.J., Eustace, A., Kidd, N., Clare, A.W., & Lawlor, B.A. (2001). Recurrent falls are associated with increased length of stay in elderly psychiatric inpatients. *International Journal of Geriatric Psychiatry, 16*, 965–968.

Hendrich, A.L. (1988). An effective unit based fall prevention plan. *Journal of Nursing Quality Assurance, 3*(1), 28–36.*

Hendrich, A.L. (1988). Unit based fall prevention. *Journal of Quality Assurance, 10*(1), 15–17.

Hendrich, A., Nyhuuis, A., Kippenbrock, A., & Soja, M.E. (1995). Hospital falls: Development of predictive model for clinical practice. *Applied Nursing Research, 8*, 129–139.

Hill, B.A., Johnson, R., & Garrett, B.J. (1988). Reducing the incidence of falls in high-risk patients. *Journal of Nursing Administration, 18* (7/8), 24–28.*

Jones, W., & Smith, A. (1989). Preventing hospital incidence. What can we do? *Nursing Management, 20* (9), 58–60.

Kilpack, V., Boehm, J., Smith, N., & Mudge, B. (1991). Using research-based interventions to decrease patient falls. *Applied Nursing Research, 4* (2), 50–56.

Lawerence, J.I., & Maher, P.L. (1992). An interdisciplinary falls consult team: A collaborative approach to patient falls. *Journal of Nursing Care Quality, 6* (3), 21–29.

Lim, K.D., Ng, K.C., Ng, S.K., & Ng, L.L. (2001). Falls amongst institutionalized psycho-geriatric patients. *Singapore Medical Journal, 42*, 466–472.

Llewellyn, J., Martin, B., Shekleton, M., & Firlit, S. (1988). Analysis of falls in the acute surgical and cardiovascular surgical patients. *Applied Nursing Research, 1*(3), 116–121.

Maciorowski, L.F., Munro, B.H., Dietrick-Gallagher, M., et al. (1988). A review of the patient fall literature. *Journal of Nursing Quality Assurance, 3* (1), 18–27.

Mayo, N.E., Korner-Bitensky, N., Becker, R., & Georges, P.C. (1989). Preventing falls among patients in a rehabilitation setting. *Canadian Journal of Rehabilitation, 2*(4), 235–240.

McCollam, M.E. (1995). Evaluation and implementation of a research-based falls assessment program. *Nursing Clinics of North America, 30*(3), 507–514.*

McFarlane, M.A., & Melora, P. (1993). Decreasing falls by the application of standards of care, practice, and governance. *Journal of Nursing Care Quality, 8*(1), 43–50.

Mion, L.C., Gregor, S., Buettner, M., et al. (1989). Falls in the rehabilitation setting: Incidence and characteristics. *Rehabilitation Nursing, 14*(1), 17–22.

Morse, J.M., Black, C., Oberle, K., & Donahue, P. (1989). A prospective study to identify the fall-prone patient. *Social Science Medicine, 28*(1), 81–86.*

Morse, J.M., Morse, R.M., & Tylko, S. (1989). Development of a scale to identify the fall-prone patient. *Canadian Journal on Aging, 8*, 366–377.*

Morton, D. (1989). Five years of fewer falls. *American Journal of Nursing, 89*(2), 204–205.

Quinlan, W.C. (1994). The liability risk of patients who fall. *Journal of Healthcare Risk Management, 14*, 29–33.

Oliver, D., Britton, M., Seed, P., Martin, F.C., & Happer, A.H. (1997). Development and evaluation of evidence based risk assessment tool (STRATIFY) to predict which elderly inpatients will fall: Case-controlled and cohort studies. *British Medical Journal, 315*, 1049–1053.

Oliver D., Hopper, A., & Seed, P. (2000). Do hospital fall prevention programs work? A systematic review. *Journal of the American Geriatrics Society, 48*, 1679–1689.

Roberts, B.L. (1993). Is stay in an intensive care unit a risk for falls? *Applied Nursing Research, 6*, 135–136.

Rohde, J.M., Myers, A.H., & Vlahov, D. (1990). Variation in risk for falls by clinical department: Implications for prevention. *Infection Control and Hospital Epidemiology, 11*, 521–524.

Ross, J.E.R. (1991). Iatrogenesis in the elderly: Contributors to falls. *Journal of Gerontological Nursing, 17*(9), 19–23.

Ruckstuhl, M.C., Marchionda, E.E., Salmons, J., & Larrabee, J.H. (1988). Patient falls: An outcome indicator. *Journal of Gerontological Nursing, 6*(1), 25–29.*

Savage, T., Matheis-Kraft, C. (2001). Fall occurrence in a geriatric psychiatry setting before and after a fall prevention program. *Journal of Gerontological Nursing, 27*, 49–53.

Schmid, N.A. (1990). Reducing patient falls: A research-based comprehensive fall prevention program. *Military Medicine, 155,* 202–207.

Spellbring, A.M. (1992). Assessing elderly patients at high risk for falls: A reliability study. *Journal of Nursing Care Quality, 6*(3), 30–35.*

Spellbring, A.M., Gannon, M.E., Kleckner, T., & Conway, K. (1988). Improving safety for hospitalized elderly. *Journal of Gerontological Nursing, 14,* 31–36.*

Stevenson, B., Mills, E.M., Welin, L., & Beal, K.G. (1998). Falls risk factors in an acute-care setting: A retrospective study. *Canadian Journal of Nursing Research, 30,* 97–111.

Tutuarima, J.A., de Haan, R.J., & Limburg, M. (1993). Number of nursing staff and falls: A case-control study by stroke patients in acute-care settings. *Journal of Advanced Nursing, 18,* 1101–1105.

Uden, G., Ehnfors, M., & Sjostrom, K. (1999). Use of initial risk assessment and recording as the main nursing intervention in identifying risks of falls, *Journal of Advanced Nursing, 29,* 145–152.

Vassallo, M., Amersey, R.A., Sharma, J.C., & Allen, S.C. (2000). Falls on integrated medical wards. *Gerontology, 46,* 158–162.

Vlahov, D., Myers, A.H., & Al-Ibrahim, M.S. (1990). Epidemiology of falls among patients in a rehabilitation hospital. *Archives of Physical Medicine and Rehabilitation, 71,* 8–12.

Way, B.B. (1992). The relationship between staff–patient ratio and reported patient incidents. *Hospital and Community Psychiatry, 43,* 361–365.

Whedon, M.B., & Shedd, P. (1989). Prediction and prevention of patient falls. *Image: Journal of Nursing Scholarship, 21*(2), 108–114.*

Zepp, S. (1991). Ban "a" fall: A nursing innovation to reducing patient falls. *Kansas Nurse, 66*(7), 13.

NURSING FACILITY

Eakman, A.M., Havens, M.D., Ager, S.J., Buchanan, R.L., Fee, N.J., Gollick, S.G., Michels, M.J., Olson, L.L., Satterfield, K.M., Stevenson, K.A. (2002). Fall prevention in long-term care: An in-house interdisciplinary team approach. *Topics of Geriatric Rehabilitation, 17,* 29–39.

Franzoni, S., Rozzini, R., Boffelli, S., et al. (1994). Fear of falling in nursing home residents. *Gerontology, 40,* 38–44.

Friedman, S.M., Williamson, J.D., Lee, B.H., et al. (1995). Increased fall rates in nursing home residents after relocation to a new facility. *Journal of the American Geriatrics Society, 43,* 1237–1242.

Ginter, S.G., & Mion, L.C. (1992). Falls in the nursing home: Preventable or inevitable? *Journal of Gerontological Nursing, 18,* 43–48.

Gross, Y.T., Shimamoto, Y., Rose, C.L., et al. (1990). Why do they fall? Monitoring risk factors in nursing homes. *Journal of Gerontological Nursing, 16*(6), 20–25.

Harris, P.B. (1989). Organizational and staff attitudinal determinants of falls in nursing home residents. *Medical Care, 27,* 737–749.

Harrison, B., Booth, D., & Algase, D. (2001). Studying fall risk factors among nursing home residents who fell. *Journal of Gerontological Nursing, 27,* 26–34.

Janitti, P.O., Pyykko, I., & Laippala, P. (1995). Prognosis of falls among elderly nursing home residents. *Aging: Clinical and Experimental Research, 7,* 23–27.

Jonsson, P.V., Lipsitz, L.A., Kelley, M., et al. (1990). Hypotensive responses to common daily activities in institutional elderly: A potential risk for recurrent falls. *Archives of Internal Medicine, 150,* 1518–1524.

Kerman, M., & Mulvihill, M. (1990). The role of medication in falls among the elderly in a long-term care facility. *Mount Sinai Journal of Medicine, 57,* 343–347.

Krueger, P.D., Brazil, K., & Lohfeld, L.H. (2001). Risk factors for falls and injuries in a long-term care facility in Ontario. *Canadian Journal of Public Health, 92,* 117–120.

Kuehn, A.F., & Sendelweck, S. (1995). Acute health status and its relationship to falls in the nursing home. *Journal of Gerontological Nursing, 21*(7), 41–49.

Lipsitz, L.A., Jonsson, P.V., Kelley, M.M., et al. (1991). Causes and correlates of recurrent falls in ambulatory frail elderly. *Journal of Gerontology, 46,* M114–M122.

Luukinen, H., Koski, K., Laippala, P., & Kivela, S.L. (1995). Risk factors for recurrent falls in the elderly in long-term institutional care. *Public Health, 109*(1), 57–65.

Micelli, D.L.G., Wasman, H., Cavalieri, T., & Lage, S. (1994). Prodromal falls among older nursing home residents. *Applied Nursing Research, 7*(1), 18–27.

Myers, A.H., Baker, S.P., Robinson, E.G., et al. (1989). Falls in the institutionalized elderly. *Journal of Long-Term Care Administration, 17*(4), 12–16.

Myers, A.H., Baker, S.P., Van Natta, M.L., et al. (1991). Risk factors associated with falls and injuries among elderly institutionalized persons. *American Journal of Epidemiology, 133,* 1179–1190.

Myers, A.H., Van Natta, M.L., Robinson, E.G., & Baker, S.P. (1994). Can injurious falls be prevented? *Journal of Long-Term Care Administration, 22* (2), 26–29, 32.

Neufeld, R.R., Tideiksaar, R., Yew, E., et al. (1991). A multidisciplinary falls consultation service in a nursing home. *Gerontologist, 31,* 120–123.

Nowalk, P.M., Prendergast, J.M., Bayles, C.M., D'Amico, F.J., & Colvin, G.C. (2001). A randomized trial of exercise programs among older individuals living in two long-term care facilities: The FallsFREE program. *Journal of American Geriatrics Society, 49,* 859–865.

Ray, W.A., Meador, J.A., Thapa, P.B., Brown, A.K., Kajihara, H.K., Davis, C., Gideon, D.G., & Griffin, M.R. (1997). A randomized trial of a consultation service to reduce falls in nursing homes. *Journal of the American Medical Association, 278,* 557–562.

Ray, W.A., Thapa, P.B., & Gideon, P. (2000). Benzodiazepines and the risk of falls in nursing home residents. *Journal of the American Geriatrics Society, 48,* 682–685.

Robbins, A.S., Rubenstein, L.Z., Josephson, K.R., et al. (1989). Predictors of falls among elderly people: Results of two population-based studies. *Archives of Internal Medicine, 149,* 1628–1633.*

Ross, J.E.R. (1991). Contributors to falls. *Journal of Gerontological Nursing, 17,* 19–23.

Rubenstein, L.Z., Josephson, K.R., & Osterweil, D. (1996). Falls and fall prevention in the nursing home. *Clinics of Geriatric Medicine, 12(4),* 881–902.

Rubenstein, L.Z., Josephson, K.R., & Robbins, A.S. (1994). Falls in the nursing home. *Annals of Internal Medicine, 121,* 442–451.

Rubenstein, L.Z., Robbins, A.S., Josephson, K.R., et al. (1990). The value of assessing falls in an elderly population. A randomized clinical trial. *Annals of Internal Medicine, 113,* 308–316.

Ruthazer, R., & Lipsitz, L.A. (1993). Antidepressants and falls among elderly people in long-term care. *American Journal of Public Health, 83,* 746–749.

Svensson, M.L., Rundgren, A., Larsson, M., et al. (1991). Accidents in the institutionalized elderly: A risk analysis. *Aging, 3,* 181–192.

Thappa, P.B., Brockman, K.G., Gideon, P., et al. (1996). Injurious falls in non-ambulatory nursing home residents: A comparative study of circumstances, incidence, and risk factors. *Journal of the American Geriatrics Society, 44,* 273–278.

Thappa, P.B., Gideon, P., Brockman, K.G., et al. (1996). Clinical and biomechanical measures of balance as fall predictors in ambulatory nursing home residents. *Journal of Gerontology, 51A,* M239–M246.

Thappa, P.B., Gideon, P., Fought, R.L., & Ray, W.A. (1995). Psychotropic drugs and the risk of recurrent falls in ambulatory nursing home residents. *American Journal of Epidemiology, 142,* 202–211.

van Dijk, P.T.M., Meulenberg, O.G.R.M., van de Sande, H.J., & Habbema, J.D.F. (1993). Falls in demented patients. *Gerontologist, 33,* 200–204.

Wright, B.A., Aizenstein, S., Vogler, G., et al. (1990). Frequent fallers: Leading groups to identify psychological factors. *Journal of Gerontological Nursing, 16(4),* 15–19.

Young, S.W., Abedzadeh, C.B., & White, M.W. (1989). A fall-prevention program for nursing homes. *Nursing Management, 20(11),* 80Y, 80Z, 80AA, 80DD, 80FF.

RESTRAINTS

Blakeslee, J.A., Goldman, B.D., Papougenis, D., & Torell, C.A. (1991). Making the transition to restraint-free care. *Journal of Gerontological Nursing, 17(2),* 4–8.

Bower, F., & McCullough, C. (2000). Restraint in acute care settings: Can it be reduced? *Journal of Nursing Administration, 30,* 592–597.

Bradley, L., & Dufton, B. (1995). Breaking free. *Canadian Nurse, 91*(1), 36–40.

Bradley, L., Siddique, C.M., & Dufton, B. (1995). Reducing the use of physical restraints in long-term care facilities. *Journal of Gerontological Nursing, 21*(9), 21–34.

Brower, H.T. (1991). The alternative to restraints. *Journal of Gerontological Nursing, 17,*18–22.

Brungardt, G.S. (1994). New guidelines for a less restrictive approach. *Geriatrics, 49,* 43–50.

Bruno, R. (1994). Policy for the people: One facility's introduction to restraint reduction. *Journal of Gerontological Social Work, 22*(3/4), 129–142.

Bryant, H., & Fernald, L. (1997). Nursing knowledge and use of restraint alternatives: Acute and chronic care. *Geriatric Nursing, 18*(2), 57–60.

Burton, L.C., German, P.S., Rovner, B.W., & Brandt, L.J. (1992). Physical restraint use and cognitive decline among nursing home residents. *Journal of the American Geriatrics Society, 40,* 811–816.

Calabrese, S., Paulic, T., Callicott, D., et al. (1992). Restraint review committee: A working model. *Perspectives, 16,* 2–6.

Capezuti, E., Evans, L., Strumpf, N., & Maislin, G. (1996). Physical restraint use and falls in nursing home residents. *Journal of the American Geriatrics Society, 44,* 627–633.

Chambers, J. (1993). Eliminating physical restraint use: Implications for practice. *Journal of Nursing Administration, 23,* 5.

Clavon, A.M. (1991). Implementation of a restraint policy: A case study. *Military Medicine, 156,* 499–501.

Conely, L., & Campbell, L. (1991). The use of restraints in caring for the elderly: Realities, consequences, and alternatives. *Nurse Practitioner, 16* (12), 48–52.

Cutchins, C.H. (1991). Blueprint for restraint-free care. *American Journal of Nursing, 91*(7), 36–42.

DeSantis, J., Engberg, S., & Rodgers, J. (1998). Geropsychiatric restraint use. *Journal of the American Geriatrics Society, 12,* 1515–1518.

Dodds, S. (1996). Exercising restraint: Autonomy, welfare and elderly patients. *Journal of Medical Ethics, 22*(3), 160–163.

Dunbar, J.M., Neufeld, R.R., White, H.C., & Libow, L.S. (1996). Retrain, don't restrain: The educational intervention of the National Nursing Home Restraint Removal Project. *Gerontologist, 36*(4), 539–542.

Dunn, K.S. (2001). The effect of physical restraints on fall rates in older adults who are institutionalized. *Journal of Gerontological Nursing, 27,* 41–48.

Eigsti, D.G., & Vrooman, N. (1992). Releasing restraints in the nursing home: It can be done. *Journal of Gerontological Nursing, 18*(1), 21–23.

Ejaz, F.K., Flomar, S.J., Kaufmann, M., et al. (1994). Restraint reduction: Can it be achieved? *Gerontology, 34,* 694–699.

Ejaz, F.K., Jones, J.A., & Rose, M.S. (1994). Falls among nursing home residents: An examination of incident reports before and after restraint reduction programs. *Journal of the American Geriatrics Society, 42*, 960–964.

Elk, S., & Ferchau, L. (2000). Physical restraints: Are they necessary? *American Journal of Nursing*, (Suppl), 24–27.

Evans, L.K., & Strumpf, N. (1989). Tying down the elderly: A review of the literature on physical restraints. *Journal of the American Geriatrics Society, 36*, 65–74.

Evans, L.K., & Strumpf, N. (1990). Myths about elder restraint. *Image: Journal of Nursing Scholarship, 22*, 124–128.

Evans, L.K., & Strumpf, N.E. (1992). Alternatives to physical restraints. *Journal of Gerontological Nursing, 18*, 5–11.

Evans, L.K., Strumpf, N.E., Allen-Taylor, S.L., et al. (1997). A clinical trial to reduce restraints in nursing homes. *Journal of the American Geriatrics Society, 45*, 675–681.

Fletcher, K.R. (1990). Restraints should be a last resort. *RN, 53*, 52–55.

Frank, C., Hodgetts, G., & Puxty, J. (1996). Safety and efficacy of physical restraint for the elderly: Review of the evidence. *Canadian Family Physician, 42*, 2402–2409.

Gilbert, M., & Counsell, C. (1999). Planned change to implement a restraint reduction program. *Journal of Nursing Care Quality, 13*, 57–64.

Guttman, R., Altman, R.D., & Karlan, M.S. (1999). Report of the council on scientific affairs: Use of restraints for patients in nursing homes. *Archives of Family Medicine, 8*, 101–105.

Hall, M., & Marr, J. (1993). Patient restraint: A new philosophy. *Leadership in Health Services, 2(4)*, 22–26, 42.

Hardin, S.B., Magee, R., Stratman, D., et al. (1994). Extended care and nursing home attitudes toward restraints. *Journal of Gerontological Nursing, 20(3)*, 23–31.

Helmuth, A.M. (1995). Nurses' attitudes toward older persons on the use of physical restraints. *Orthopedic Nursing, 14(2)*, 43–51.

Hennessy, C.H., McNelly, E.A., Whittington, F.J., et al. (1997). Perceptions of physical restraint use and barriers to restraint reduction in a long-term care facility. *Journal of Aging Studies, 11(1)*, 49–62.

Janelli, L.M. (1995). Physical restraint use in acute care settings. *Journal of Nursing Care Quality, 9(3)*, 86–92.

Janelli, L.M., Dickerson, S.S., & Ventura, M.R. (1995). Nursing staff's experiences using restraints. *Clinical Nursing Research, 4(4)*, 425–441.

Janelli, L.M., Kanski, G.W., & Neary, M.A. (1994). Physical restraints: Has OBRA made a difference? *Journal of Gerontological Nursing, 20*, 17–21.

Janelli, L.M., Scherer, Y.K., Kanski, G.W., & Neary, M.A. (1991). What nursing staff members really know about physical restraints. *Rehabilitation Nursing, 16*, 345–349.

Janelli, L.M., Scherer, Y.K., Kuhn, M.M., et al. (1994). Acute/critical care nurses' knowledge of physical restraints. *Journal of Nursing Staff Development, 10*, 6–11.

Johnson, S.H. (1990). The fear of liability and the use of restraints in nursing homes. *Law, Medicine and Health Care, 18,* 263–273.

Johnson, S.H. (1991). Nursing home restraints: The legal issues. *Health Progress, 23,* 18–19.

Karlsson, S., Bucht, G., Eriksson, S., & Sandman, P. (2001). Factors relating to the use of physical restraints in geriatric care settings. *Journal of the American Geriatrics Society, 49,* 1722–1728.

Kallmann, S.L. (1992). Comfort, safety, and independence: Restraint release and its challenges. *Geriatric Nursing, 13*(3), 143–148.

Kane, R.L., Williams, C.C., Williams, T.F., et al. (1993). Restraining restraints: Changes in a standard of care. *Annual Review of Public Health, 14,* 545–584.

Kapp, M.B. (1992). Nursing home restraints and legal liability. *Journal of Legal Medicine, 13,* 1–32.

Kow, J., & Hogan, D. (2000). Use of physical restraints in medical teaching units. *Canadian Medical Association Journal, 162,* 1–3.

Leger-Krall, S. (1994). When restraints become abusive. *Nurse, 24,* 55–56.

Levine, J.M., Marchello, V., & Totolos, E. (1995). Progress toward a restraint-free environment in a large academic nursing facility. *Journal of the American Geriatrics Society, 43,* 914–918.

Lofgren, R.P., MacPherson, D.S., Granieri, R., et al. (1989). Mechanical restraints on the medical wards: Are protective devices safe? *American Journal of Public Health, 79,* 735–738.

Lusis, S. (2000). Update on restraint use in acute care settings. *Plastic Surgical Nursing, 20,* 145–150.

MacPherson, D.S., Lofgren, R.P., Granier, R., et al. (1990). Deciding to restrain medical patients. *Journal of the American Geriatrics Society, 38,* 516–520.

Magee, R., Hyatt, E.C., Hardin, S.B., et al. (1993). Institutional policy: Use of restraints in extended care and nursing homes. *Journal of Gerontological Nursing, 19*(4), 31–39.

Martin, L.S., & Huges, S.R. (1993). Using the mission statement to craft a least-restraint policy. *Nursing Management, 24*(3), 65–66.

Master, R., & Marks, S.F. (1990). The use of restraints. *Rehabilitation Nursing, 15,* 22–25.

Mayhew, P.A., Christy, K., Berkebile, J., Miller, C., & Farrish, A. (1999). Restraint reduction: Research utilization and case study with cognitive impairment. *Geriatric Nursing, 20,* 305–308.

Mercurio, A.T., & Mion, L.C. (1992). Methods to reduce restraints: Process, outcomes, and future directions. *Journal of Gerontological Nursing, 18,* 5–11.

Miles, S.H., & Irvine, P. (1992). Deaths caused by physical restraint. *Gerontologist, 32,* 762–766.

Mion, L.C., Fogel, J., Sandhu, S., Palmer, R.M., Minnick, A.F., Cranston, T., Bethoux, F., Merkel, C., Berkman, C.S., & Leipzig, R. (2001). Outcomes following physical restraint reduction programs in two acute care hospitals. *Journal on Quality Improvement, 27,* 605–618.

Mion, L.C., Frengley, J.D., Jakovicic, C.A., et al. (1989). A further exploration of the use of physical restraints in hospitalized patients. *Journal of the American Geriatrics Society, 37*, 949–956.

Mion, L.C., Strump, N., & Fulmer, T. (1994). Use of physical restraints in the hospital setting: Implications for the nurse. *Geriatric Nursing, 15*(3), 127–134.

Minnick, A., Mion, L., Leipzig, R., Lamb, K., & Palmer, R.M. (1998). Prevalence and patterns of physical restraint use in the acute care setting. *Journal of Nursing Administration, 28*, 19–24.

Morse, J.M., & McHutchion, E. (1991). The behavioral effects of releasing restraints. *Research in Nursing and Health, 14*, 187–196.

Neufeld, R.R., Libow, L.S., Foley, W., & White, H. (1995). Can physically restrained nursing-home residents be untied safely? Intervention and evaluation design. *Journal of the American Geriatrics Society, 43*, 1264–1268.

Newbern, V.B., & Lindsey, I.H. (1994). Attitudes of wives toward having their elderly husbands restrained. *Geriatric Nursing, 15*, 135–138.

Patterson, J.E., Stumpf, N.E., & Evans, L.K. (1995). Nursing consultation to reduce restraints in a nursing home. *Clinical Nurse Specialist, 9*(4), 231–235.

Phillips, C., Hawes, C., & Fries, B. (1993). Reducing the use of restraints in nursing homes: Will it increase costs? *American Journal of Public Health, 83*(3), 342–348.

Quinn, C.A. (1993). Nurses' perceptions about physical restraints. *Western Journal of Nursing Research, 15*, 148–162.

Rader, J. (1991). Modifying the environment to decrease the use of restraints. *Journal of Gerontological Nursing, 17*, 9–13.

Rader, J., Semradek, J., McKenzie, D., & McMahon, M. (1992). Restraint strategies: Reducing restraints in Oregon's long-term care facilities. *Journal of Gerontological Nursing, 18*(11), 49–56.

Registered Nurses' Association of Nova Scotia. (1995). Position statement on the use of physical restraints. . . approved by the RNANS Board of Directors, April 12, 1995. *Nurse to Nurse, 6*(3), 19.

Rodgers, S. (1994). Reducing restraints in a rehabilitation setting: A safer environment through team effort. *Rehabilitation Nursing, 19*, 274–276.

Scherer, Y.K., Janelli, L.M., Wu, Y.B., & Kuhn, M.M. (1993). Restrained patients: An important issue for critical care nursing. *Heart and Lung, 22*, 77–83.

Schirm, V., Gray, M., & Peoples, M. (1993). Nursing personnel's perceptions of physical restraint in long-term care. *Clinical Nursing Research, 2*, 98–110.

Schnelle, J.F., MacRae, P.G., Simmons, S.F., et al. (1994). Safety assessment for the frail elderly: A comparison of restrained and unrestrained nursing home residents. *Journal of the American Geriatrics Society, 42*, 586–592.

Schnelle, J.F., Newman, D.R., White, M., et al. (1992). Reducing and managing restraints in long term facilities. *Journal of the American Geriatrics Society, 40*, 381–385.

Shugrue, D.T., & Larocque, K.L. (1996). Reducing restraint use in the acute care setting. *Nursing Management, 27(10)*, 32H, 32J, 32L, 32O.

Simmons, S.A., Schnelle, J.F., MacRaie, P.G., et al. (1995). Wheelchairs as mobility restraints: Predictors of wheelchair activity in nonambulatory nursing home residents. *Journal of the American Geriatrics Society, 43*, 384–388.

Sloane, P.D., Papougenis, D., & Blakeslee, J.A. (1992). Alternatives to physical and pharmacologic restraints in long-term care. *American Family Physician, 45*, 763–769.

Stolley, J.M. (1995). Freeing your patients from restraints. *American Journal of Nursing, 95(2)*, 26–31.

Stolley, S.M., King, J., Clarke, M., et al. (1993). Developing a restraint use policy for acute care. *Journal of Nursing Administration, 23*, 49–54.

Strumpf, N.E., Evans, L.K., Wagner, J., et al. (1992). Reducing physical restraints: Developing an educational program. *Journal of Gerontological Nursing, 18*, 21–27.

Sullivan-Marx, E.M. (1994). Delirium and physical restraints in hospitalized elderly. *Image: Journal of Nursing Scholarship, 26*, 295–300.

Sullivan-Marx, E.M. (1995). Psychological responses to physical restraint use in older adults. *Psychosocial Nursing, 33(6)*, 20–25.

Sullivan-Marx, E.M. (1996). Restraint-free care: How does a nurse decide? *Journal of Gerontological Nursing, 22(9)*, 7–14.

Sundel, M., Garrett, R.M., & Horn, R.D. (1994). Restraint reduction in a nursing home and its impact on employee attitudes. *Journal of the American Geriatrics Society, 42*, 381–387.

Thomas, A., Redfern, L., & John, R. (1995). Perceptions of acute care nurses in the use of restraints. *Journal of Gerontological Nursing, 21(6)*, 32–38.

Tinetti, M.E., Liu, W., & Ginter, S.F. (1992). Mechanical restraint use and fall-related injuries among residents of skilled nursing homes. *Annals of Internal Medicine, 116*, 369–374.

Tinetti, M.E., Liu, W., Marottolil, R.A., et al. (1991). Mechanical restraint use among skilled nursing facilities: Prevalence, patterns and predictors. *Journal of the American Medical Association, 265*, 460–471.

Wells, C.F., Brown, D., & McClymount, A.A. (1994). Development of a least restraint program—one hospital's experience. *Perspectives, 18*, 10–13.

Werner, P., Cohen-Mansfield, J., Braun, J., et al. (1989). Physical restraint and agitation in nursing home residents. *Journal of the American Geriatrics Society, 37*, 1122–1126.

Werner, P., Cohen-Mansfield, J., Koroknay, V., & Braun, J. (1994). Reducing restraint: Impact on staff attitudes. *Journal of Gerontological Nursing, 20(12)*, 19–24.

Werner, P., Koroknay, V., Braun, J., & Cohen-Mansfield, J. (1994). Individualized care alternatives used in the process of removing physical restraints in the nursing home. *Journal of the American Geriatrics Society, 42*, 321–325.

Wilson, E.B. (1996). Physical restraint of elderly patients in critical care: Historical perspectives and new directions. *Critical Care Nursing Clinics of North America, 8*(1), 61–70.

SIDE RAILS

Braun, J.A., & Capezuti, E. (2000). Siderail use and legal liability issues in nursing homes. *Illinois Bar Journal, 88*, 34–6, 8–9, 32, 34.

Capezuti, E., Talerico, K.A., Strumpf, N., & Evans L. (1998). Individualized assessment and intervention in bilateral siderail use. *Geriatric Nursing, 19*, 322–330.

Feinsod, F.M., Moore, M., & Levenson, S.A. (1997). Eliminating full-length bed siderails from long-term care facilities. *Nursing Home Medicine, 5*, 257–263.

Gallinagh, R., Slevin, E., & McCormack, B. (2000). Side rails as physical restraints; the need for appropriate assessment. *Nursing Older People, 13*, 20–25.

Hager, H.C. (1999). An analysis of falls in the hospital: Can we do without bedrails? *Journal of the American Geriatrics Society, 47*, 529–531.

Hammond, M., & Levine, J.M. (1999). Bedrails: Choosing the best alternative. *Geriatric Nursing, 20*, 297–300.

Jehan, W. (1999). Restraint or protection? The use of bedside rails. *Nursing Management, 6*, 9–13.

Parker, K., & Miles, S. (1997). Deaths caused by side rails. *Journal of the American Geriatric Society, 45*, 797–802.

Si, M., Neufeld, R., & Dunbar, J. (1999). Removal of bed rails on a short-term nursing home rehabilitation unit. *The Gerontologist, 39*, 611–615.

Talerico, K., & Capezuti, E. (2001). Myths and facts about side rails. *American Journal of Nursing, 101*, 43–48.

index

ORDER ADDITIONAL COPIES OF FALLS IN OLDER PEOPLE!

ORDERING INFORMATION

Please send me _____ copies of *Falls in Older People* at $25.95 each.

Price may be higher outside U.S. Price subject to change without notice.

Shipping & Handling: For purchases of $0–$49.99, add $5; $50–$399.99, add 10% of product total; $400 and up, add 8% of product total

❏ Check enclosed (payable to Health Professions Press)
❏ Purchase order (purchase order must be attached)
❏ Credit card: ___ MasterCard ___ VISA ___ American Express

Card no. _____ Exp. date _____

Signature _____

Name _____

Institution _____

Street Address _____

_____

City/State/ZIP _____

Daytime phone (____)_____

This address is (check one):
❏ Residential ❏ Commercial

HEALTH PROFESSIONS PRESS   PO BOX 10624
BALTIMORE, MD 21285-0624
TOLL-FREE: 888-337-8808
FAX: 410-337-8539 • PHONE: 410-337-9585
www.healthpropress.com

**FOR INFORMATION ON QUANTITY DISCOUNTS,
CONTACT OUR CUSTOMER SERVICE DEPARTMENT** 3TD